Health Care, Technology, and the Competitive Environment

Health Care, Technology, and the Competitive Environment

EDITED BY
Henry P. Brehm and **Ross M. Mullner**

677274

PRAEGER

New York
Westport, Connecticut
London

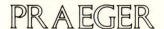

Library of Congress Cataloging-in-Publication Data

Health care, technology, and the competitive environment / edited by
  Henry P. Brehm and Ross M. Mullner.
    p. cm.
  Based in part on papers presented at a conference sponsored by and
held at the Center for Technology and Policy, Boston University,
Sept. 1987.
  Bibliography: p.
  ISBN 0-275-93033-5 (alk. paper)
  1. Medical technology—United States—Congresses. 2. Medical
care—United States—Congresses. I. Brehm, Henry P. II. Mullner,
Ross M. III. Boston University. Center for Technology and Policy.
  [DNLM: 1. Biotechnology. 2. Delivery of Health Care—economics—
United States. 3. Delivery of Health Care—trends—United States.
4. Economics, Hospital—United States. 5. Technology, High-Cost.
WX 157 H43445]
R855.2.H43   1989
610'.28—dc20   89–3961

Library of Congress Catalog Card Number: 89–3961
ISBN: 0-275-93033-5

First published in 1989

Praeger Publishers, One Madison Avenue, New York, NY 10010
A division of Greenwood Press, Inc.

Printed in the United States of America

The paper used in this book complies with the Permanent
Paper Standard issued by the National Information Standards
Organization (Z39.48–1984).

10 9 8 7 6 5 4 3 2 1

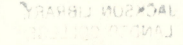

To Our Wives,
Molly and Linda

Contents

Figures and Tables

TABLES

Preface

There have been major advances in diagnostic and therapeutic technology over the past several years that have changed care delivery approaches within the U.S. health system. These care approaches differentially impact the cost of care and the financial position of traditional providers.

Technological developments in an earlier time period, including anesthesia, antiseptic techniques, X-ray procedures, and antibiotics, made it possible to perform more-sophisticated medical procedures in the hospital and were the basis for the hospital emerging as the center for complex patient care. Modern technological developments have added high points of sophistication to the health care arsenal but have also made it possible to do more on an outpatient basis and to shorten hospital lengths of stay.

Advances in technology have been responsible for a major part of the increased cost of medical care; nonlabor expenses have risen significantly as a percentage of total hospital expenses. This has contributed to the double pressure to reduce both the cost and the use of inpatient care.

The change in Medicare from a cost-based retrospective reimbursement program to a Prospective Payment System using diagnosis-related groups (DRGs) directly affects reimbursement for a major share of the hospital market. Additionally, hospitals have been facing an increasingly competitive environment, with declining admissions, average daily censuses, and occupancy rates. Alternative delivery systems and settings increase the competitive pressures. Concerns for the rising costs of health care and their share of the gross national product provide added pressure on the health care delivery market. This increased competition and concern for the cost of care also impact the implementation of technological developments.

The change under Medicare did not alter the system to make it financially beneficial for hospitals to reduce the need for hospitalization. Hospitals do not receive Medicare or other insurance payments for empty beds. As a result, keeping the beds occupied is a major focus of concern. Maintaining state-of-the-art technology can serve that purpose. However, innovative health care technology may or may not hold the promise of being cost reducing for a given episode of hospitalization initially or at any time in the future. Its cost benefit may rest in reduced need for future care or improved productive capacity of the patient. The hospital's technology decision-making will ignore cost effects at the risk of its own financial situation. The general implications for future innovation in health care and development of health care technology cannot be ignored.

In September 1987, the Center for Technology and Policy, Boston University, sponsored a conference entitled: "Health Technology Adoption in a DRG Age." The conference focused on how the change in Medicare's hospital reimbursement approach and the increased competitiveness in the health care delivery market altered the balance of factors affecting decisions on adoption and diffusion of given types of biomedical technology. The center, as the university's focal point for the study of technology strategy and policy issues, was the appropriate locus for a discussion of the interplay between technology and the changed environment in which health care is delivered, an issue with implications for the future of biomedical technology innovation.

The present volume is based only in part on papers presented at the September 1987 conference. Many of the chapters were not part of the conference; some papers given at the conference are not included in this book. However, the conference served as the inspiration for developing the original theme into this book.

The coeditors express their appreciation to Dr. Gerald Gordon, then Director of the Center for Technology and Policy, and to the center and Boston University for their assistance in making the conference and this book a reality. We would also like to thank Seragen, Inc., and Karl Ahrendt, Chief Executive Officer, for the financial support provided for the conference. A special note of thanks goes also to Nancy Gordy for her efforts in putting this book together.

Health Care, Technology, and the Competitive Environment

1

Introduction: The Changing Scene in Hospital Care

Henry P. Brehm and Ross M. Mullner

Few observers could have predicted the changes that have taken place in hospital care within the past several years. Technological advances had altered the content and approach of health care as well as the settings for its delivery. Alongside this, modifications in the organization, delivery, and financing of health care that would have seemed at best improbable 10 years ago and impossible 30 to 40 years ago have irrevocably changed the nature of American health care.

When the Hill-Burton Act was passed in 1946 with the objective of promoting the development of increased bed capacity in U.S. hospitals, who could have expected that we would reach a point of declining hospital admissions along with pressure to reduce excess bed capacity? How many years ago was it that the administrator of a hospital viewed other hospitals in the area as parts of a cooperative inpatient care network rather than as potential competitors? Hospitals did not compete for market share nor did they advertise their services. Neither were they concerned about the possible detrimental effects on themselves as business entities of sharing information and resources with neighboring facilities. The concern was for patient care and improving the quality of that care; "business" concerns occupied a lower order of priority.

In the years since 1946 we have moved through three distinct eras in governmental efforts to affect the availability, accessibility, and affordability of health care facilities and services. The first era, as reflected in the Hill-Burton Act, was one of promoting expansion. This approach basically was maintained through the early years of the Medicare and Medicaid programs. In the early 1970s, in response to what was seen as unacceptable increases in the use and cost of health care services with their impact on the federal budget, the medical care component of the consumer price index, and the percentage of the gross national product devoted to health care, we moved to an era of efforts to control these issues by regulation.

In the 1980s the focus changed to one of attempting to raise cost-consciousness among providers and users of health care services as well as among the third-party payers for these services. The intent was to effect cost control by heightening competition among providers in the industry and shifting more payment responsibility back to the user population. The era of cost control and use control through increased competition was expected to make users and those who paid for managed care more prudent consumers and to make providers more sensitive to the impact of cost control and efficiency on their financial situation.

The primary focus in providing hospital care is still on the quality of patient care, but the circumstances under which that care is provided and the pressures for cost control and resource management have been radically altered. The business end of running a hospital has become a more significant consideration. That does not mean that all decisions now made in hospitals are based solely on the financial best interests of the organization and not on the care needs of the patients served, but clearly there are pressures in this direction.

CHANGES IN HOSPITAL REIMBURSEMENT AND ORGANIZATION

Hospital admissions, average daily censuses, and occupancy rates have been decreasing, creating market pressures to fill empty beds. Alternative delivery systems and settings have increased the level of competition within the traditional hospital's market. Concerns for the cost of care and its share of the gross national product have increased these pressures within the health system.

The restructuring of Medicare and, more recently, the limitations on periodic adjustments in the program's payment levels in combination with the increased competition in the health care marketplace have heightened concerns for the business end of providing hospital care. They have increased the pressures for cost-consciousness and control.

Medicare introduced the Prospective Payment System (PPS) using diagnosis-related groups (DRGs) in 1983 as part of an attempt to control rapidly rising costs in the health care industry. The changed approach for reimbursing hospitals for the inpatient care of beneficiaries eliminated cost-based retrospective reimbursement in favor of prospective payment for care based on the DRG into which the patient is classified. This was a major alteration in how Medicare pays for hospital services. The change was to be phased in over several years, directly affecting reimbursement for a large share of the hospital market. As originally designed, the 467 DRGs were determined from a set of 23 major diagnostic categories, further differentiated by whether the case was a surgical or medical one, the specific procedure performed, the patient's age, and the presence or absence of complications and comorbidities (Office of Technology Assessment, 1985).

A different payment schedule was established for urban and rural hospitals. However, no differentiation in payment was provided for by the type of hospital, with referral centers receiving the same amount as all other hospitals. The assumption was that since the DRG system is a case-mix approach, the increased severity of cases treated in referral hospitals would be reflected in higher dollar values for the DRGs handled and, as a result, higher total reimbursement to such hospitals from Medicare. Additionally, the system was designed to work on the understanding that losses on some cases would balance out against gains on others.

The hospital receives the same payment per DRG (with a minor exception for outliers limited to 5–6% of cases) regardless of how long the patient stays or the actual cost of the care provided. If the cost of care administered by the hospital exceeds the DRG level, the full cost no longer can be recovered and the hospital has to absorb the loss. However, if the DRG payment exceeds the cost of care, the hospital can keep the excess. The system was designed to provide an incentive to hospitals for cost efficiency. Under the old mechanism a hospital received reimbursement for the cost of providing inpatient care as long as such care was medically justified and accepted under utilization-review procedures.

The move to the PPS was made in the expectation that it would favor cost-reducing technologies and contribute to an overall reduction in health care costs. In practice, this has not happened yet. However, experts are beginning to worry that a new cost-consciousness among health care providers may force them to think twice about adopting and using new lifesaving technologies with a large price tag. The new environment in the health care system results in pressures to economize.

Corporate restructuring of hospitals has been a common phenomenon in recent years. A variety of benefits can derive from the hospital's being a part of a larger corporate entity, whether a multihospital chain or a single hospital within a more complex corporate structure. It permits separating various activities and services from the direct operation of the hospital, reducing their involvement with regulatory and accrediting agencies. For example, the not-for-profit hospital activities can be put in a unit independent of any for-profit ventures, fund-raising and development planning efforts, or similar activities that are necessary to the organization but not part of the hospital's care mission. A larger corporate structure also can make various resources and services such as financial planning or bulk purchasing more readily available to the individual hospital than would otherwise be the case.

ORGANIZATION OF THE CHAPTERS TO FOLLOW

This volume focuses on how these changes in the hospital environment have altered the balance of factors affecting adoption and diffusion decisions for given types of biomedical technology. The chapters are divided into four sections.

Part I, Technology and Health Care Content, reviews developments and the state of the art within various categories of medical technology and biotechnology and the implications for patient care content and approaches, the settings for care delivery, and patient recovery, longevity, and others. It considers the relationship between technology and care delivery and care-delivery capacity in the modern hospital and in alternative-care settings.

Part II, Technology and the Health Care Organization, reviews technology decision-making and the information base used in that process within industrial concerns and how this has differed from the medical setting. It deals with the factors affecting such decision-making within hospitals and the effect this has on technology development, adoption, and use, and at the interplay of technology with organizational structure, staffing, and financial position of the provider organization.

Part III, Technology and the Changing Environment, reviews the changes affecting technology development and adoption. It looks at the changes in hospital reimbursement, primarily under Medicare, and their significance for recovering expenditures related to technology development and adoption and at the changes in the nature of the health care market as these interrelate with technology.

Part IV, Implications for Technology Policy, discusses the conclusions that can be derived from this collected work. It considers the implications for technology development and adoption, for the financing of technology and health care provision, and for health care organization and delivery.

PART I
TECHNOLOGY AND HEALTH CARE CONTENT

2

Categories of Medical Technology

Stan N. Finkelstein

To approach the topic of categories of medical technology, I turn to three different perspectives on the issues and problems facing medical technology, one written in the early 1970s, another in the mid–1970s, and the last in the early 1980s. These three essays reflect an evolution in thinking about the directions, priorities, and trends that were ongoing in this field.

The phrase *medical technology* refers to a broad definition that includes most practices and products in use in health care, diagnosis, prevention, or rehabilitation. It includes equipment-embodied technology but also takes in methods, procedures, and software. In this chapter I will concern myself with medical rather than managerial applications of technology.

AN EARLY–1970s PERSPECTIVE

The author of the first essay is Lewis Thomas, former dean of the Yale University School of Medicine and retired president of the Memorial Sloan Kettering Hospital and Cancer Institute in New York. For many years he has written "Notes of a Biology Watcher," a column that appears periodically in the *New England Journal of Medicine* (Thomas, 1974). In 1971 he published a piece in that column entitled "The Technology of Medicine." He principally argues that whatever the main problems facing medical technology, present or future, recognized or unanticipated, the ultimate solution is to encourage medical research that will elucidate the underlying mechanisms of important diseases.

Through this elucidation effective treatments and solutions to distribution problems will emerge.

Thomas presented a scheme that divided the technology of medicine into three categories: nontechnology, halfway technology, and the genuine technologies of medicine. Of those three the one that has been most widely repeated is halfway technology. Thomas began by reflecting that technology assessment had become by the 1970s relatively routine outside of health with vast sums of money being spent on such things as economic impact analysis of space and defense research. As of 1971 the technology of medicine had been largely taken for granted by these kinds of analysts. In medicine, the major problem with technology has been, in Thomas's view, the need to stimulate development and access to that development. He predicts that advocates of technology assessment will eventually discover a medical battlefront and is concerned that they keep separate what he views to be fundamentally different kinds of medical technology.

Nontechnology was his first category, which he describes as the caring and support offered to patients with disease problems that we do not understand at all and cannot do much of anything about, but for which we have to do something. Among the examples he offered were the therapeutic approaches to infectious diseases that were around in the early part of the 20th century before the relatively recent advances in antibiotics and immunizations, and also before progress in public health caused the reversal and in many cases the virtual elimination of those diseases. He points out that the support that was needed for them was not particularly technical in nature, yet they were very cost-intensive, hospital-intensive, and physician time- and skill-intensive. Yet, ultimately there was little to show for it.

One of his examples could have been the iron lung, used to treat polio before more effective preventions and treatments emerged. Its use was very costly in its time and had little or no effect on the course of the disease. However, a recently published article by James Maxwell (1986) reported a historical case study of the iron lung and found that it does not really qualify under Thomas's definition of nontechnology. Maxwell documented a number of innovations that eventually emerged from the iron lung that have had an impact on modern medical practices.

Thomas's second category, the one with which many people are familiar, is halfway technology. In his view, halfway technology represents the kind of practices that must be done, often after the fact, in efforts to compensate for the incapacitating effects of certain diseases that we can do something about, but not much. Halfway technology that potentially postpones death includes organ transplantation and renal dialysis. Thomas argues that we are content to postpone death—to extend life—because we are not yet able to reverse the process of destruction of the kidney at the cellular and molecular level. He would argue that if we knew enough about the mechanism of the disease, we could introduce new technologies to reverse it.

Cancer chemotherapy is another example of a halfway technology. One of the principles of some cancer chemotherapy is that the agents are highly toxic to many normal and diseased cells but are especially active against cells in the dividing stage. As part of this therapy, many normal cells must be killed—not just cancer cells. But the idea is that since cancer is largely a disorder of cell division, at any given time there are more cancer cells dividing than normal ones and that more cancer cells are destroyed. Thomas would argue that if we knew the mechanisms of the underlying disorders we were dealing with, the superior approach would be to reverse the disease. Halfway technology, he says, is at the same time highly sophisticated and profoundly primitive. We resort to it because of a lack of understanding of the mechanisms of disease, and very possibly it must be done until something better comes along.

Thomas's final category was what he called the genuine technology of medicine—effective but attracting the least public notice. Immunization and antibiotics are among the most prominent examples that he identified. He argues that genuine technology comes about as the result of a real understanding of the disease mechanisms. The technology that emerges is so obviously inexpensive and effective that there is little need to take the trouble to conduct a cost-benefit analysis or similar study. He hopes that policy analysts who are going to advocate and conduct these assessments in health will not divert funds from medical research and slow the understanding of disease processes that will lead to more genuine technologies.

A MID–1970s VIEW

A few years later, Howard Hiatt published an article entitled "Protecting the Medical Commons: Who Is Responsible?" (Hiatt, 1975). Hiatt, former chief of medicine at Beth Israel Hospital and former dean of the Harvard School of Public Health, is a scholar of medicine and health policy. Hiatt argues that (as of when he wrote this paper) there was now a need to conduct the kind of technology assessments and evaluations that Thomas predicted would come to be done in the health field. Hiatt also wanted to make certain that physicians play a part in that process.

Hiatt's article on the medical commons was based in part on an earlier piece by population biologist Garret Hardin (1968). Hardin's argument refers to the consequences of uncontrolled population growth on the resources available to society. He writes:

The tragedy of the commons develops in this way. Picture a pasture open to all. It is to be expected that each herdsman will try to keep as many cattle as possible on the commons. Such an arrangement may work reasonably satisfactorily for centuries because tribal wars, poaching and disease keep the numbers of man and beast well below the carrying capacity of the land. Finally, however, comes the day of reckoning, that is, the day when the long desired goal of social stability becomes a reality. At this point, the inherent logic of the commons remorselessly generates tragedy. As a rational being each herdsman seeks to maximize his gain, explicitly or implicitly, more or less consciously he asks, ''What is the utility to me of adding one more animal to my herd?'' This utility has one negative and one positive component. The positive component is a function of the increment of one animal since the herdsman receives all the proceeds from the sale of the initial animal, the positive utility is plus one. The negative component is a function of the additional overgrazing created by one more animal. Since, however, the effects of overgrazing are shared by all the herdsmen, the negative utility for any particular decision-making herdsman is only a fraction of minus one.

Adding together the component partial utilities, the rational herdsman concludes that the only sensible course for him to pursue is to add another animal to the herd, and another, and another. But this is the conclusion reached by each and every rational herdsman sharing the commons, and therein is the tragedy; each man is locked into a system that compels him to increase his herd without limit in a world that is limited.

Hiatt wanted to draw a parallel about the constraints on a society delivering health care. He writes:

The total resources available for medical care can be viewed as analogous to the grazing area on Hardin's commons and the practices drawing on those resources to Hardin's grazing animals. Surely nobody would quarrel with the proposition that there is a limit to the resources that any society can devote to medical care and few would question the suggestion that we are approaching such a limit.

Recall that Hiatt wrote those words in 1975 when the percentage of the GNP devoted to health care was under 8%. It is now around 11%.

Hiatt argues that if one is to take steps to avert the tragedy of the commons in health care, careful consideration must be given clinical evaluation and technology assessment in three particular categories where he believes resources could ultimately be conserved: medical practices reflecting individual versus society conflict; those in common use yet having either no value or undetermined value; and medical practices applied to potentially preventable conditions.

Individual versus Society Conflict

There are a number of disorders that have a very low frequency, where the costs of identifying those afflicted with the disorder can be extremely high, but once identified and treated, particular individuals can do really well. The problem lies in the observation that frequency of occurrence can be so low that cost-effectiveness from society's vantage point might not be high. An example often given to illustrate this phenomenon is a newborn screening problem for the metabolic disorder phenylketonuria (PKU), an enzyme deficiency in phenylalanine metabolism in which the body lacks the enzyme to convert one amino acid to another, and as a result there is a buildup of intermediate products toxic to the central nervous system. There are tests that can be administered at birth, and those with positive tests can be effectively treated with diet. Not long ago, screening programs for PKU were mandated by most states. Some states no longer mandate the screening program because costs of those programs are high and the frequency of occurrence rate is quite low.

Medical Practices of No Value or Undetermined Value

A large number of medical practices are in current use despite either evidence that they have little value, or little evidence that they have value. Some of those practices are holdovers from an earlier time when our capabilities to evaluate technology were much less than they are now. As an illustration of the problem, it is useful to point out that for many years a common treatment for a wide range of disorders involved bleeding patients to rid their systems of the causative agents of disease. After World War II came the development and widespread civilian use of blood transfusion to compensate for certain conditions that deplete one or another blood component. Much more recently, many practitioners have resumed the use of sophisticated bleeding techniques to filter potentially noxious substances from the circulation. It can be argued that the presence or absence of evaluative data on the effectiveness of these procedures neither greatly helped nor hindered their adoption.

Medical Practices for Potentially Preventable Conditions

A good example comes from the research of David Eddy, a physician and mathematician from Duke University, who wrote the award-winning *Screening for Cancer* (Eddy, 1980). Eddy looked systematically at the research literature evaluating alternative treatments for a number of different forms of cancer. He assembled and interpreted the literature and arrived at recommendations that emerged from logical and systematic thinking applied to these problems. Partly on the basis of Eddy's work, the American Cancer Society changed some of its long-standing recommendations on the frequency of having certain tests that screen for cancer. One change in particular was to lengthen the recommended interval for a chest X ray from once every six months to much less frequently than that. Why? The essence of the argument is that if cancer of the lung comes to diagnosis because of symptoms—cough, hoarseness, or spitting up blood— the average life expectancy from diagnosis could be around one and one-half years. On the other hand, if the lung cancer had been diagnosed by chest X ray, it comes to attention on average one and one-half years earlier than it does from symptoms, at which time average life expectancy may be around three years. During those three years there is ample time for a wide range of costly inter- ventions including major surgery that on a statistical basis may not favorably impact either the length or quality of life. Hiatt's argument here might be that the cost effectiveness of lung cancer diagnosis and treatment may not be as favorable as that of an educational program or other public campaign to reduce cigarette smoking.

Hiatt advocated increasing use of evaluation of this sort and wanted to assure that physicians were not left out of the process. Thomas had correctly predicted that someone of Hiatt's stature in the medical field would soon strongly advocate technology assessment.

A 1980s Perspective

A third and final view that I will discuss emerged from a project on biomedical innovation, in which I participated, sponsored by the National Heart, Lung, and Blood Institute of NIH and the Sloan School of Management at MIT (Roberts et al., 1981). Our work suggests that as we move increasingly to evaluate medical technology that it be done in such a way to preserve the future development of innovation in the health field. As we wrote,

Since the Second World War, the biomedical field has simultaneously experienced an information explosion and remarkable technical advances in the detection, diagnosis, therapy, rehabilitation, and the prevention of disease. Today very highly sophisticated technology is available for some problems; but for others, technology is either inadequate or nonexistent. The development and dissemination of medical practices has not always occurred in an optimal fashion. Some efficacious medical practices have been adopted too slowly; some practices have been displaced too slowly; and others, though clinically valuable, have been too costly.

A logical inference from this work would be to ask whether some categories of technologies in the medical care area have been net-cost reducing and others net-cost raising. Some of my colleagues involved in the biomedical innovation project had experience evaluating work in electronics and computers applied to defense and space needs. They have argued that much of the innovation that eventually took place in these fields was process innovation, usually associated with a reduction in costs. But it has been frequently suggested that in the health care field little cost-reducing technological innovation has taken place.

With the emergence of prospective payment and other financial constraints, technology assessment (a phrase that does not have a standard meaning and each user may intend a different connotation) is now being advocated or conducted by myriad government agencies, professional societies, insurance carriers, and other organizations.

The cost of medical technology has in a number of instances determined how its manufacturers are promoting it. Some years ago I was invited, along with a cohort of academic colleagues from Boston, to a conference held in a Florida resort organized by a university under contract from a drug company and called "National Conference on Cost-Benefit Analysis: 'Product C' as a Model." "Product C," not identified by name in this chapter, is a best-selling drug to prevent and treat a common gastrointestinal disorder in adults. When our group of academics arrived at this conference we were surprised to find that in addition to other university colleagues invited to share research findings on the use of cost-benefit analysis in medical technology evaluation, others in attendance included the formulary managers of many of the Medicaid programs from states around the country. By coincidence or not, a number of the invited papers suggested by inference that Product C was favorably regarded in these cost-benefit analyses. A possibly worrisome extension of this trend would be if manufacturers were strictly to gear their product development to the payment system. A colleague who recently returned from an industry trade association meeting in Washington said he heard the phrase *product design for reimbursement* used more than once. If that becomes a watchphrase of our medical product innovation, then we may truly have reasons for concern.

In this chapter I have contrasted three essays that offer their own categories of medical technology. Thomas's essay predicts pessimistically that technology assessment would come to medicine, and his categories help anticipate what the analysts will find. A few years later, Hiatt advocated technology evaluation in medicine and offered his typology of categories in which he believed it would prove beneficial. And more recently, the article from *Biomedical Innovation* implies that a cost-reducing category of innovation in medicine should be possible and attention needs to be paid simultaneously to both evaluating medical technology and stimulating its development. Despite the problems it may have directly or indirectly created, medical technology is one large reason the American health delivery system is strong. Appropriate actions ought to be taken to see that it remains that way.

3

Biotechnology and Health Care: The Potential Impact on Care Content, Approaches, and Settings

James P. Sherblom

For a decade now, much has been written about the coming cornucopia of biotechnology products and the impact they will have on health technology. In the last 10 years alone, more than $5 billion has been spent by companies trying to develop health care products utilizing this new technology. And yet to date, the combined share of the U.S. health care dollar spent on biotechnology products is miniscule. This chapter will outline briefly the current status of development of biotechnology products and their likely impact on the health care industry, including care content, settings, and financing.

Biotechnology is the application of modern biology as a tool in man's continued search for improved health care, food, and other agricultural products. It often involves the application of new biological techniques to traditional health care problems; but it seldom, if ever, involves anything quite as esoteric as the popular press would like us to believe. The principles of biotechnology were first applied to human health care, through the use of living organisms, as early as 5000 B.C. for the creation of early medicine. The properties of certain plants and herbs were often employed in the form of medicinal extracts. The bark of the cinchora tree, for example, is still used today to make quinine, an important drug in the treatment of malaria.

Living organism were and still are today used to change flour into bread, grape juice into wine, and milk into cheese. Of course these early uses of biotechnology were discovered by trial and error, or accident, generally without an understanding of the scientific principles involved. An important breakthrough

Table 3.1
Biotechnology Health Care Products Already on the Market

	Expected Market Size U.S. 1990 ($ millions)	Expected FDA Approval
Human Insulin	125	On Market
Human Growth Hormone	100	On Market
Alpha Interferon	100	On Market
Hepatitis B Vaccine	100	On Market
Monoclonal Antibodies	300	On Market
TOTAL	$725 million	

Source: Kidder Peabody Biotechnology Analyst (Peter Drake: personal communication).

came in the 19th century when Gregor Mendel discovered the principles of heredity. His studies of several generations of pea plants and the resulting theories helped to lead to the modern era of biotechnology.

Over the next 100 years, scientific knowledge about the laws of heredity rapidly accumulated and climaxed with the proof that deoxyribonucleic acid, better known as DNA, is the source of genetic information in all living things. With an understanding of the structure and role of DNA, it became apparent that the crude improvements in plants and animals over the previous centuries had been accomplished by hit-or-miss genetic manipulations. Scientists then began the task of altering DNA with understanding and precision under carefully controlled conditions. It is this skill that we call biotechnology. It has opened up tremendous advances in the field of medicine and human health care that promise to change the way we think about treating diseases.

A number of biotechnology products have come on to the market in the last two years and are projected to represent very sizable markets by 1990. Projections made by Peter Drake, Kidder Peabody's biotechnology analyst for human insulin, human growth hormone, alpha interferon, hepatitis B vaccine, and various monoclonal antibodies suggest that these products alone could represent U.S. sales of $725 million by 1990 (see Table 3.1). These products are being produced utilizing a number of new techniques and are making plentiful and relatively cheap substances that were formerly extremely rare and, hence, very expensive. The real increase in new products, however, will come from the introduction of products over the next three years that are currently in clinical trials. T-PA (tissue plasminogen activator), Interleukin 2, and Erythropoietin are all expected to

Table 3.2
Biotechnology Health Care Products Expected to be Introduced by 1990

	Expected Market Size U.S. 1990 ($ millions)	Expected FDA Approval
Tissue Plasminogen Activator		
(t-PA)	400	1988
Interleukin-2	200	1988
Erythropoietin	150	1988
Factor 8	100	1989
Epidermal Growth Factor	100	1989
Colony Stimulating Factors	100	1989
Other New Therapeutics	150	1989-90
TOTAL	$1.2 billion	

Source: Kidder Peabody Biotechnology Analyst (Peter Drake: personal communication).

receive FDA approval in 1988. Factor 8, epidermal growth factor, a number of colony stimulating factors, and various smaller drugs are expected to receive approval by 1990 (see Table 3.2). The introduction of these new drugs along with the growth of those already on the market could expand biotechnology's contribution to human therapeutics in the United States to $2 billion annually by 1990.

The general press writes frequently and quite extensively about the potential promise of new drugs such as t-PA and Interleukin 2. These are very exciting drugs and certainly represent the largest near-term market for biotechnology products. And, as you would expect, their enormous potential is reflected in the fact that there are six to eight biotech firms earnestly at work to introduce various competitive forms of each of these drugs. What is not obvious from the general literature, however, is that these blockbuster products represent only the tip of the iceberg. Perhaps more important in considering biotechnology's overall impact on human health care will be the larger number of biotechnology products developed to treat smaller, less common diseases. Each of these products typically is developed by one firm only, addresses a relatively small market, and is virtually ignored by the business and financial press. However, each of these products is a significant breakthrough for the patients it will treat, many of whom were often untreatable previously, and collectively these products address a relatively large segment of the health care market.

One product with which I am intimately familiar serves as an example of the potential impact of this new technology. Gaucher's disease is a rare genetic disease that results in an enlarged liver and spleen, bone erosion and fractures, as well as severe anemia. There are fewer than 20,000 Gaucher's patients in the United States, and up until now their disease has been for all practical purposes untreatable. The disease, however, often makes their lives quite miserable. Genzyme Corporation has, in collaboration with the National Institutes of Health over the last 10 years, developed a successful treatment for Gaucher's disease that will be commercially available in 1989. This drug is expected to significantly reduce the symptoms of the disease and, hence, measurably improve the quality of patients' lives. This disease would have remained untreatable but for the advances in modern biology. Several drugs of this nature, though individually representing small markets, are estimated by Peter Drake to equal total markets of $150 million by 1990. Collectively they will probably over the long term have a larger effect on human health care than t-PA alone.

However, let us return for brevity's sake to a discussion of the impact of biotechnology's major products. The availability of t-PA and similar products will change the way we treat heart disease. Recombinantly produced Erythropoietin and Factor 8 will dramatically improve our ability to treat blood disorders. Products scheduled to become available over the next few years, e.g., the interferons, interleukins, and tumor necrosis factor, should significantly increase our ability to treat cancer patients. More importantly, the understanding of cancer we are gaining in attempting to develop and improve these products is dramatically advancing our understanding of how this disease functions and advances.

New vaccines will also allow us to control diseases at an earlier stage. Examples of vaccines currently under development at biotechnology firms include vaccines for AIDS, hepatitis B, malaria, and herpes. Each of these vaccines could significantly reduce the spread of these communicable diseases. Other improvements in our capabilities to diagnose cancer and infectious diseases will result from products coming into the market over the next two years (see Table 3.3). It is foreseeable that with genetic screening it will one day be possible to predict and prevent higher-risk candidates from contracting cancer, and if they are stricken, to diagnose and treat the cancer at a very early stage.

So what will be the likely impact of all these new biotechnology products on care content, settings, and financing? I believe that we will be able to vaccinate against more diseases and hence slow their spread through the population as well as diagnose the disease in patients at an earlier and less-costly stage. This could mean fewer people contracting diseases, and less-severe cases when the disease is contracted. This ought to allow us to treat more patients on a doctor-office or outpatient basis. And for those who must be hospitalized, it could mean shorter and less-critical hospital stays with a reduced requirement for surgical intervention. All of these advances would represent improvements in care content and reductions in costs per patient to treat particular diagnosis-related groups (see Figure 3.1).

However, the biotechnology products themselves are the result of years of extremely expensive research and development followed by very extensive clin-

Table 3.3
Diagnostic Biotechnology Products Currently Available or Soon to be Released

	Expected Market Size U.S. 1990 ($ millions)	Expected FDA Approval
Infectious disease detection	80	On Market
Hepatitis B diagnosis	40	On Market
AIDS	75	On Market
Cancer blood tests	100	1987
Cancer imaging	75	1987
Cardiac imaging	50	1988
TOTAL	$420 million	

Source: Kidder Peabody Biotechnology Analyst (Peter Drake: personal communication).

Figure 3.1
Likely Impact of Biotechnology on Health Care

o   Better quality of life

        -Vaccines (hepatitis B, malaria, herpes, AIDS)

        -Early detection/diagnosis

        -Less-invasive treatment

o   More congenial treatment setting

        -At home

        -Doctor's office/outpatient

o   A change in the structure of patient costs

        -Higher drug costs

        -Lower overall costs per patient

ical trials prior to FDA approval. The average research cost of a product per patient treated will of necessity be much higher for biopharmaceuticals than for traditional chemical pharmaceuticals. These costs will have to be recouped through higher per-patient drug costs. As a result, in most cases biotechnology products will be quite expensive compared to previous drugs.

In summary, what we can expect from this influx of new biotechnology products is a reinforcement of trends already occurring in U.S. health care. The availability of vaccines and the capability of early detection and diagnosis of diseases should lead to a better quality of life for most patients. The doctors of those hospitalized will have available a wider variety of less-invasive treatment approaches. These new approaches are ideal candidates for outpatient or doctor-office applications, and in some cases will even be self-administered by the patient at home. Drug costs are likely to increase as the result of these biotech-nological products, but the overall cost of patient care should decline markedly.

In this chapter I have limited myself for brevity's sake to expected new products over the next few years. Naturally, as we look out toward the year 2000, the expected impact of biotechnology on human health care is far greater and should extend to the treatment of numerous other disease groups. To date we have only seen the first fruit of a cornucopia of potential new products that will increasingly influence human health technology during the remainder of this century.

4

Technological Innovations and Their Impact on Care Delivery

Joyce Grahl Riley and Henry P. Brehm

Major technological innovations over the last several years have changed patient care approaches within the U.S. health system. While such innovations bring to mind machines with shiny chrome and flashing lights, the U.S. Office of Technology Assessment uses a much broader definition in determining the boundaries of health care technology. It includes devices, but also pharmaceuticals and biologics, the medical and surgical procedures used in medical care, and the organizational and support systems with which such care is delivered. The devices run the gamut from ultracomplex, capital-intensive equipment to consumable or disposable items used in patient care. In *Medicine and Its Technology*, technology is described as an intermediary between science and mechanics (Davis, 1981). Whether a broad or narrow view of medical technology is used, it would take superhuman ability to keep up with all new technology as it is introduced. Health care providers are challenged just to keep up with changes in their own specialties.

As new technology is incorporated into the health system, it impacts on the delivery of care, more so for some items than for others. One of the most obvious effects is when new technology changes the care setting. There was a time when almost all sick care was given in the home. Family members, persons skilled in healing, and later, trained physicians rallied to the patient's bedside and provided what was available in the way of diagnosis, treatment, and care. Hospitals were seen as a last resort and then only for the poor who had no family or resources to be cared for at home.

By the late 1800s, two separate technological advances helped change this attitude: the development of antiseptic procedures and the use of general anesthesia. These, along with the later advent of antibiotics, combined to improve the tolerance for and outcomes of surgical procedures. It became clear that the hospital was the best place to perform surgery. The environment could be more easily controlled, and all of the equipment and personnel needed would be on hand.

By the 1900s, much of the technology being developed was concentrated in hospitals which became more and more important in the delivery of health care. There was a rapid growth in medical technology that escalated during and following World War II. The war produced advances in the development of antibiotics and new techniques for the treatment of trauma and burns (Torrens, 1988).

Physicians began to divide their time between the office and the hospital. Home visits, while still made, were not encouraged by the physician; these went from 10% of all ambulatory physician visits in 1958 to 1% in 1974 (Sidel & Sidel, 1983). Meanwhile, consumers were being educated to the concept that physicians could better serve them in the office or hospital where all the "tools" needed to establish a diagnosis or provide treatment were located.

The hospital became a technological center. Most equipment was too expensive for individual physician practices to support. Doctors expected the latest innovations to be available to them as part of their hospital attending privileges. Hospitals wanted the latest technology to attract and maintain a roster of good physicians. This would also help hospitals establish reputations for excellence in the communities they served. A permissive third-party reimbursement system not only allowed but encouraged inpatient use of services for anything from a diagnostic test to a major surgical procedure.

While technological innovation has affected industry in general, its impact on the health system as an industry appears somewhat different. In the health system, most technology is process technology, i.e., technology used within an industry to produce a product. In this case the product is health care. This is not conceptually different from various manufacturing industries where innovative process technology is used in manufacturing technologically advanced products. The critical distinction in how technology relates to the health system is that health care is not the system's end product but is itself a process used to reach the desired end product, health or wellness. Using innovative process technology to produce the next stage of process technology is not unique within the health system, but it does result in potential strains on the system.

New process technology has substantially improved the product within various service industries from banking and financial advising to home entertainment and shopping. In some ways the situation in the health system is similar. The desired end product is changing because of the effect of process technology.

Health care delivery's focus on innovations in diagnostic technology where the necessary therapeutic technology still does not exist marks it as different from other industries. This is an emphasis on process technology that does not as yet lead to an improvement in the end product. This is found acceptable based on the need to improve diagnosis before effective treatment is possible.

The biomedical technology and biotechnology industries produce a major share of the products used as the process technology within health care delivery. They are affected by the demands of users and final consumers in the health system for new and improved technology. In other industries the competitive consuming market for both process and product technology is expected to be a restraining factor limiting the development and diffusion of innovations with high cost relative to benefit. In health care, can we expect the same from the patient or the patient's family as the ultimate consumer, or from those who use the process technology in delivering care?

If we accept health or wellness as the end product of the health system, we need to define it in terms that are operationally relevant for health care delivery. Should the primary focus be on the continuation of life, or should this be pursued only if an acceptable minimal quality of life is possible? Technological advances in health care have intensified the life quantity/quality debate by permitting providers to do more in both areas. These advances also have changed our expectations in both areas.

In the area of health and, therefore, in the areas of health care and health care technology, we are immediately faced with serious legal, moral, and social considerations centering on the issue of defining the end product. This is not the case relative to other areas of process technology and their impact on the product. Certainly there are legal issues regarding the delivery of banking services or the protection of consumer rights that may affect or be affected by a technological advance. If this happens, the application of the technology can be restrained or delayed pending resolution of the issue. However, there is no driving force of a continuous requirement to do more beyond the push to improve competitive position. In health care there is a moral requirement to do more embodied in the standards of the provider professions, and incorporated, to some degree, into the legal requirements to continue care once started.

However, technology that permits you to do more than could be done previously may increase, not decrease, the overall cost of care. It may substantially improve the ability to diagnose, treat, or even prevent disease or to rehabilitate patients and restore lost functional capacity. It may well delay the inevitability of death for patients for whom there is no reasonable prospect of return to an acceptable quality of life.

Additionally, as advances in process technology come on line and extend the quantity of life, this can result in greater demand for the use of existing technology and for the development of more, and more expensive, process technology. The end product is health, but the lack of a clear definition for this end product creates more of a moving target than in other industries. Therein lies the dilemma of the end product of care and the function of technology within the care process.

The technology revolution has affected the cost of care, particularly in hospitals, and raised concerns about cost control and efficiency. It also has provided opportunities for out-of-hospital care, reducing the need for inpatient care and increasing competition among hospitals for patients. This raises the following issues: How does technology affect health care content and settings? What financial pressures are hospitals facing from competition and reimbursement changes particularly as these relate to technology? Within this changing environment, how "business like" are hospitals in their behavior towards the adoption and use of technology?

Today the trend is to reduce the amount of time the patient spends in the hospital. Technological innovations have decreased the number of inpatient days required for many treatments and in some cases eliminated the need for hospitalization altogether. Technological developments have increased the range of care services that can be provided to patients, have broadened the definition of treatable conditions, and have simplified the treatment of certain conditions. This last factor has made it possible to treat an increasing number of patients in alternative-care settings and as outpatients who previously would have needed services available only on an inpatient basis.

Few technological innovations in health care fall in the category of new and less expensive processes for producing the same or a similar product. Some developments are clearly in this category, and they potentially can impact care settings and costs, e.g., percutaneous transluminal coronary angioplasty (PTCA), and arthroscopic and laser surgery. These technologies have, for patients for whom their use is appropriate, reduced the cost of care as well as eliminated the need for more complex surgical procedures. However, they have not replaced the more complex procedures available for health care, but rather added to the existing structure. As a result, while they have reduced the cost for specific care procedures, they have not reduced the overall costs of the health system.

The flexibility afforded health care by technology innovations has contributed to changes in the organizational structure and settings for care delivery. Not-for-profit hospitals used to virtually control the domain of inpatient care. They now are increasingly under pressure from the for-profit hospitals that operate a growing percentage of total hospital beds in this country (American Hospital Association [AHA], 1987). For-profit facilities sometimes find it advantageous to specialize in a single form of care for uncomplicated cases, removing a share of the market for potentially more profitable cases from not-for-profit acute care general hospitals. Advances in surgical procedures and aftercare also enable surgicenters to treat patients who previously would have been treated as inpatients.

Under the pressure of competition for a declining inpatient market from alternative-care settings and from other hospitals, some hospitals have attempted to broaden the range of their marketability by providing more ambulatory care and by offering community outreach services for health or wellness maintenance. Hospitals increasingly are positioning themselves to expand or contract specific services based on their market expectations and the image as a care facility they wish to present to the user community.

TECHNOLOGY AND REIMBURSEMENT APPROACHES

Technology alone does not account for changes in patterns of use of inpatient hospital services. Just as a permissive reimbursement system can foster use of inpatient services, a restrictive system can discourage the use of these services. Demands by third-party payers and group health insurance managers for more cost-conscious use of health resources play an important role in the decrease in hospital use. Third-party payers have responded to the opportunities afforded by the new technology available by either requiring that some procedures not be performed on an inpatient basis or by giving the provider an incentive not to do so. In those circumstances where these procedures are being used in treatment, this has reduced the demand for hospital beds and contributed to the heightened competition among hospitals for the remaining candidates for inpatient care.

As a result, the average number of discharges from nonfederal short-stay hospitals has been on a steady decline since 1981, dropping from 160.2 per 1,000 population to 132.8 in 1986 (Public Health Service, 1987). This, coupled with a continuing decrease in the average length of stay, indicates a reduction in use of inpatient services.

The most obvious example of increased pressure for cost-consciousness among third-party payers is the 1983 Medicare change to a Prospective Payment System (PPS) for inpatient hospital services. This change was part of an effort by the federal government to influence trends in the development and use of technology by making the major institutional provider, the hospital, more cost conscious. In combination with the technological developments themselves, these changes have reduced the demand for inpatient care.

While the Medicare change was being put in place, traditional health insurance programs began more universally to require approval for nonemergency hospital admissions, second opinions for elective surgery, and for certain diagnostic and surgical procedures to be routinely done on an outpatient basis. However, third-party payers are only able to make these demands because medical technology is available that permits patients to be treated safely and effectively in this manner.

Under the old Medicare hospital payment approach, retrospective reimbursement based on cost, the standard industry model, new technology could be justified if it would be of some benefit to the patient. Assuming a certificate of need (CON) could be obtained as well as the up-front financing, any additional cost involved in caring for the patient could be recovered through the reimbursement system. Since Medicare patients, primarily those 65 and over, use about 35–40% of the inpatient care received in this country, this was a significant issue for technology decisions.

Under the PPS, new care technology that increases the cost relative to reimbursement may lower the profitability of such care. If the full cost of care is no longer being recovered, this may produce an operating loss for the hospital.

While capital improvement costs are not yet included under the DRGs (see Mullner, Chap. 15), operating costs for new technology are. Much new technology in the health arena, particularly in the early stages, results in a higher, not a lower, cost of caring for the patient. For any new technology considered, the lack of cost benefit may seriously impede its adoption. Similarly, this situation could limit the expansion in use of unprofitable technology.

As an added layer of complication, there is an interchange between new technology and the DRG classification system and mechanisms for its periodic adjustment. How a given technology is coded as a procedure and how it is treated when the relative prices of DRGs are recalibrated can affect its profitability. Also, how technology-based quality enhancements are accounted for in the annual update of DRG prices can have a financial impact on technology in general.

These changes in the reimbursement approach could affect the way the hospital behaves relative to decision-making for the adoption of new technology or for expansion in the use of existing technology. The general pressure is for cost-reducing technologies, unless it is possible to justify a higher DRG payment level because of the care advances the new technology affords.

Where previously the decision on adoption and use of technology could be based primarily on quality of care issues, it now must be sensitive to the effect of technology on cost of care and reimbursement potential. Different technologies have different implications for investment cost, cost of administration, use of personnel, length of hospital stay, reimbursement through other than the DRG mechanism, outpatient use potential, and related items that affect the total cost of care and the ability to recover these costs.

The rise of managed care programs, including health maintenance organizations (HMOs) and preferred provider organizations (PPOs), has put additional limitations on the hospital (National Committee for Quality Health Care, 1987). Managed care programs, which now control some 5% of the health care business, can contract with designated hospitals and specify what and how much care is to be provided under prescribed conditions and what the level of reimbursement will be (Egdahl, 1987). The effect of such programs is that new and updated technology will be purchased in competition with nursing salaries, new and renovated facilities, and other hospital budgetary items in a more managed environment.

The interplay between technology and the changed environment in which health care is delivered has implications for the future of biomedical technology innovation. The clearest issue in the current health care delivery scene is that technology decision-making must consider factors in addition to quality of care. Technology adoption and diffusion decisions need to deal with the realities of a drastic alteration in a major reimbursement program and the impact of a competitive market. Reimbursement and competition differentially affect different types of technology with varying cost, use, and outcome potentials. The complexities of technology policy and strategy and the interplay among kinds of technology and organization, staffing, and finance issues now should be increasingly important in decision-making.

TECHNOLOGY AND CARE SETTINGS, DELIVERY, AND PROVIDERS

Taking into account this background of the relationships between technology and health care, we can now consider some specific technologies and their interactions with the system. Arthroscopic surgery is an example of how technology has reduced hospital use in the treatment of knee injuries. Such injuries have been a problem for pro and amateur athletes. Prior surgical treatment often required a long recovery period. The new approach allows knee repairs to be done through a small incision and does not disrupt the uninvolved anatomy of the joint. The recovery time is measured in days or weeks rather than months (Easterbrook, 1987).

New imaging devices such as the CT scanner and magnetic resonance imager (MRI) provide information that eliminates the need for some exploratory diagnostic surgery. Scans can be done on an outpatient basis. Thus, during the diagnostic phase of care, the necessity for hospitalization is reduced. This is a frequent result of new diagnostic and therapeutic technology.

Hospitals themselves are providing facilities for outpatient surgery. Some of these surgicenters are annexed to the hospital; others have been developed as freestanding facilities in communities some distance from the owner-hospital. Surgical procedures such as cataract removal, hernia repairs, tissue biopsies, and more are routinely performed in these centers. The patients arrive early the morning of the scheduled procedure, having already received outpatient preparation for the operation. Following surgery, they are monitored while recovering from anesthesia, and are checked for any complications resulting from the procedure. The length of time the patient is monitored depends on the procedure performed and the patient's response. Patients are released with appropriate post-op instructions and medications, often getting home in time for lunch.

The first of these surgicenters was established in 1970 (Wilson & Neuhauser, 1985). Initially, these were opened by physicians or physician group practices, some specializing in a specific type of surgery such as cosmetic procedures. The recent trend has been towards development by hospitals.

Physicians have set up facilities to provide outpatient diagnostic and therapeutic services in other areas that would normally be carried out in hospital settings. Radiologist groups have purchased CT scanners and other therapeutic and diagnostic technology. They provide services on a referred outpatient basis. Other physician groups have opened walk-in treatment clinics. The "doc-in-the-box," as it has become known, offers the community an alternative to the hospital emergency room for the treatment of non-life-threatening injuries and illnesses.

New technology has made the patient's home a viable alternative care setting again. Implantation of an infusion pump for controlled release of therapeutic drugs not only reduces hospitalization time but also allows the patient to continue the treatment process at home. The pump is designed to be surgically implanted below the surface of the skin and can be refilled externally. In this way, chemotherapy can be administered directly to a specific site or a specific blood level of medication, e.g., insulin or pain medication, can be maintained. A nurse or technician can visit the patient at home and report the patient's progress to a physician (Easterbrook, 1985; Office of Technology Assessment, 1985).

However, new technology has not overcome the need for a primary care giver in the home environment in some situations. This responsibility is usually expected to fall on the patient's personal support network. When such support is not available, home health care may not be feasible.

The continual development and diffusion of technology into the delivery system not only affects care settings but also fosters the specialization of care providers. As innovations in instrumentation and equipment were introduced for use in diagnosis and treatment, physicians began to specialize in the study and care of specific organ systems. Ophthalmology was one of the early medical specialties (Davis, 1981).

More recently, nursing also has established practice specialties in order to define more clearly and fulfill its place in the changing health care delivery system. Nurse practitioners are RNs who have completed additional training to prepare them for expanded roles and responsibilities. There are pediatric, nurse midwife, family, adult, psychiatric, and geriatric nurse practitioner programs (Moscovice, 1988).

Additionally, new technology has been a major factor in the development of specialized health occupations (Department of Health and Human Services [DHHS], 1984). As of 1984, 141 different allied health occupations were identified (Bruhn & Philips, 1985). Even though there continues to be an increase in the physician-to-population ratio, the ratio of physicians to other health care workers is decreasing. At the turn of the century, 1 out of 3 health care workers was a physician. By the early 1980s, physicians only represented 1 out of every 16 health workers (Aries & Kennedy, 1986).

As the advent of new equipment and devices made the provision of care more complex, duties that had been performed by physicians and nurses were now shared or taken over by new specialized provider occupations. For example, radiologic health services has experienced an expansion with the developments of ultrasound scanning, computerized tomography, and magnetic resonance imaging. In addition to radiologists, medical specialists, there are radiographers, nuclear medicine technologists, and radiation therapy technologists, all providing patient services (DHHS, 1984).

The development of more-sophisticated life-support equipment and treatment modalities of the cardiopulmonary system has created specialized workers to assist in the provision of care. Respiratory therapists and respiratory therapy technicians set up, operate, and monitor equipment designed to assist patients with breathing. Perfusion technologists operate the heart-lung machine used for cardiopulmonary bypass during surgery (DHHS, 1984; AHA, 1982).

This does not even scratch the surface of the number and variety of technologists, therapists, and technicians who are active in patient care. Most of the educational and training programs were established during or after 1970, and many have gone through an accreditation or approval process (DHHS, 1984).

A complicating factor in new technology's effect on care settings and staffing is that such development does not always mean the replacement of existing techniques in the provision of care. As technology is diffused into the delivery system, the result may be that more options are provided for the care giver and receiver. Sometimes new technology allows additional, different care for the same condition, an increase in care intensity. Other times it gives diagnostic or treatment alternatives for conditions, creating the need for selective evaluation. Nowhere can the add-on of new technology to existing technology be seen more clearly than in the field of diagnostic imaging.

The X ray was discovered by Roentgen in 1895. By the early 1900s it was being used as a diagnostic tool. In time, the equipment was refined, reducing risk of exposure to X radiation and improving the quality of the image produced. Additional diagnostic procedures were developed and imaging further improved by the injection of contrast agents into vessels, body cavities, and tissues.

During the mid–1970s, a new approach to diagnostic imagery exploded into the health care scene, the computed-axial tomograph, or CT scanner. Here was the ultimate in diagnostic imaging. Every hospital had to have one, hang the cost; almost all did. It did reduce the need for exploratory surgery and scoping procedures. Because of the large number manufactured to meet the system's demand, the cost dropped considerably.

Just as the industry was catching its breath from the advent of the CT scanner, the early 1980s heralded yet another wonder machine, the MRI. This uses a strong magnetic field instead of ionizing radiation to create an image. It also provides a better picture, reduces the need for contrasting dyes, and requires little patient preparation. Because calcium emits no MR, it can image tissues surrounded by bone that are difficult to study by CT scanning ("Magnetic Resonance Imaging," 1988).

Each of these innovations in imaging technology has influenced the delivery of care by adding to the physician's ability to diagnose more accurately. Collectively, this technology area has reduced the need for surgery and the pain and risk to the patient. When more-invasive treatment is needed, the physician is better prepared by the information provided.

However, the more recent imaging innovations have not completely replaced the earlier technology in the physician's plethora of diagnostic devices. Flat-plate X rays are still taken routinely for screening and diagnostic purposes; the MRI has not replaced the CT scanner as the ultimate imaging tool. Each is used separately and in conjunction with the others for clarifying and further defining the diagnosis.

There is evidence that when more is available to do to the patient, more is done. The American Hospital Association uses an intensity index that measures 37 hospital inputs provided per patient-day. These measures include lab tests,

X rays, prescriptions, visits to the operating room, and nursing person-hours. Between January 1970 and October 1979 the intensity index rose 55%. One study indicted that approximately 39% of the increase of cost per patient-day could be attributed to more intense use of selected medical services. Another study following a large, multispeciality, fee-for-service physician practice between 1951 and 1971 found that the average number of laboratory tests for a ruptured appendix went from 5.3 to 31.0. The average number of tests for maternity care almost tripled; five times as many tests were being done for breast cancer (Goldfarb et al., 1980).

TECHNOLOGICAL INNOVATIONS: DESCRIPTIVE EXAMPLES

A variety of health care innovations are of interest because of their influence on the range of treatable conditions and patient outcomes, as these interact with the selection of treatment options and care settings. Technology's interaction with reimbursement because of the changed Medicare approach also is an issue of concern. In this regard, the Office of Technology Assessment (OTA) reviewed, as of 1985, how a series of emerging technologies potentially could both affect and be affected by the change under Medicare to a PPS approach (OTA, 1985). The interest here is on how the DRG payment levels and the mechanisms for setting and adjusting them can affect the adoption or abandonment of technology.

The PPS was never intended to affect uniformly the range of medical technologies (OTA, 1985). However, it was expected in general to encourage the development and diffusion of cost-saving technologies and to discourage the use of cost-raising ones. It should have provided incentives for the adoption and use of technologies that decreased per-case operating costs compared to alternatives; increased admissions for simple procedures in profitable DRGs, including those that otherwise might have been done on an outpatient basis; or, were highly visible, benefiting the hospital's image so that it would attract admissions and fill beds. In the area of decreasing per-case operating costs, this could happen because the technology lowered lengths of stay, was less labor intensive, permitted fewer or less-frequent ancillary services, or was a supply technology that lowered costs. Additionally, the adoption and use of a new technology, even a cost-increasing one, could be encouraged if this permitted patient classification, by procedure code assignment, into a higher-paying and more profitable DRG than was previously the case. However, a new technology that reduced per-case cost could injure the hospital financially if its use placed the patient in a lower paying DRG (OTA, 1985).

In general, the interaction problems between emerging technologies and the PPS relate to the distinction between lower-paying medical DRGs and higher-paying surgical ones and to the use of the procedure codes in the International Classification of Diseases, Ninth Revision, Clinical Modifications (ICD–9–CM) as a basis for payment. The ICD–9–CM codes were designed for clinical and statistical purposes. Information on the current treatment of these technologies under the PPS, where provided, was obtained in discussions with OTA, HCFA, or the Prospective Payment Assessment Commission (ProPAC) staff.

A variety of technological innovations that have emerged in the last several decades could be discussed in detail for their impact on the health care system. Obviously, this chapter is not the appropriate format for such a comprehensive review. However, some specific examples of such technological innovation will be discussed, including a range of laser applications in health care, PTCA, and extracorporeal shock wave lithotripsy (ESWL).

Lasers

Lasers can be used in patient care as a less-invasive technique than traditional surgical approaches. The word *laser* is actually an acronym for *light amplification by stimulated emission of radiation*. "Lasers produce an intense beam of light of uniform wavelength and color that can be precisely focused to deliver high levels of energy to small areas" (Joffe & Schroder, 1987, 125).

The first laser was produced and described in July 1960 by T. H. Maiman of the Hughes Aircraft Laboratories (Hertzberg, 1986). This was a ruby laser. Since then, other types of lasers using different mediums have been developed. Medicine uses various lasers for different applications (e.g., carbon dioxide, Nd:YAG, ruby, argon, tunable dye, and excimer) (JAMA, 1986).

Because of the variety of focused light beams generated and the various operating modes, different lasers are used for different purposes. An early use of the laser was for photo coagulation of blood. The laser can be used effectively in surgery as a cutting tool and to vaporize tissue selectively. More recently, treatment procedures have been developed using lasers after making tissues selectively photosensitive. This increases the effectiveness of lasers for destroying targeted tissue, such as cancer cells (Council on Scientific Affairs, 1986).

Ophthalmology was the first specialty to embrace the use of lasers. By 1963, treatment had moved from experimental animals to human patients (Geyer & Lazar, 1986). The ruby laser was found useful in sealing retinal holes. Today, the ophthalmic surgeon can use laser technology to coagulate, vaporize, ablate, and cut eye tissue with less invasive, and less traumatizing methods than those previously used (Geyer & Lazar, 1986; Haik, Terrell & Haik, 1987). Use of lasers has advanced treatment and therefore improved outcomes for many ophthalmic conditions. One area in which laser techniques are especially effective is in the treatment of glaucoma. The laser iridotomy nonsurgically creates a shunt for the treatment of narrow-angle glaucoma. Other laser procedures are effective in treating primary and advanced open-angle glaucoma (Haik, Terrell & Haik, 1987).

Laser therapies are also useful in treating selected cases of diabetic retinopathy, macular degeneration, retinal tears and detachment, and as a follow-up procedure for cataract surgery. Laser ophthalmic procedures reduce risk of infection, need for hospitalization, need for general anesthesia, and recovery time and discomfort experienced by the patient. New uses are continuing to be developed and refined (Geyer & Lazar, 1986; Haik, Terrell & Haik, 1987).

Gynecology is probably second only to ophthalmology in the surgical use of lasers. Laser vaporization is a treatment for cervical cancer (intraepithelial neoplasia). Follow-up studies show cure rates ranging from 76% to 97%. It can be performed on an outpatient basis with local or no anesthesia. Laser coinization of the cervix, in selected cases, can be used in place of the cold knife. It has the advantage of reduced bleeding and reduced risk of stenosis following the procedure. In addition to cervical cancer, the laser is effective in the treatment of vaginal and vulvar neoplasia. It is also helpful in treating venereal warts (condylomax acuminata). Gynecological applications of laser endoscopy, particularly the treatment of endometriosis, and intraabdominal laser surgery show promise as effective care modalities (Baggish, 1986; Council on Scientific Affairs, 1986).

Other medical specialties have incorporated laser therapies into their treatment arsenal. Oncology uses lasers in the palliative treatment of carcinomas of the gastrointestinal tract. They are used with an endoscope to relieve obstruction and as a result often prolong life (Joffe & Schroder, 1987; Council on Scientific Affairs, 1986). Lasers are effective in treatment of cancer of the head (including mouth and tongue) and neck, often with less trauma and disfigurement to the patient, and improved healing (Aronoff, 1986).

Successful treatment of various benign and vascular tumors is accomplished by laser therapy (Aronoff, 1986). They are helpful in controlling bleeding from a variety of lesions such as peptic ulcers. Urologists find lasers effective in the fragmentation of some urinary tract stones, prostatectomy, and partial nephrectomy, and see promise in treating bladder cancer with photodynamic therapy. There are laser applications in plastic surgery and dermatology from simple removals of birthmarks and tattoos to treatment of extensive skin cancer. Lasers are also used to reattach traumatized limbs, fingers, and toes (Joffe & Schroder, 1987).

This is by no means an all-inclusive survey of the uses of lasers in medicine. It does give some indication of the variety of ways they have been incorporated into medical care. New applications are continuing to be developed, and we are probably still a long way from stretching the limits of the uses of lasers in delivering health care.

Percutaneous Transluminal Coronary Angioplasty (PTCA)

The development of new technology for treating coronary artery disease requires an evaluative process through which the physician must select the treatment option for this condition that best suits the patient. Heart disease is the leading cause of death in the United States. Lifestyle changes could reduce or eliminate much of the risk of coronary heart disease. For those who do succumb to coronary arteriosclerosis today, there are treatment alternatives. The one that has been around the longest is a regime of diet, exercise, and medication. This is still the treatment of choice for some patients. However, many severely impaired are not helped by this therapy.

Advanced cases may need more invasive techniques: bypass surgery or PTCA. Bypass surgery provided a real breakthrough alternative for those previously not relieved by medical treatment. It allowed people who would otherwise have been crippled by their disease to live active, productive lives. In this surgery, the blocked coronary artery is "bypassed" by a grafted healthy vessel usually taken from the patient's leg. In PTCA, the coronary artery is opened by passing a catheter with an inflatable balloon. These treatment modalities may be used individually or in combination with each other. PTCA is the more recent technological development in the treatment of coronary arteriosclerosis. This balloon dilatation procedure was developed by Andreas Gruentzig in 1974 (Baim, 1988) and became viable as a treatment procedure in the late 1970s. Its use has increased and broadened considerably over time.

Initially, less than 20% of patients requiring revascularization were considered eligible for PTCA (Reeder et al., 1984). A more recent study of 50 physician operators experienced in angioplasty indicated that today more than 50% of those referred for revascularization are being treated with PTCA (Baim & Ignatius, 1988).

Over time, further development of equipment and technique and increased operator training and experience have improved outcomes of the procedure. This was evidenced in a study of PTCA cases registered with the National Heart, Lung, and Blood Institute (Detre et al., 1988). The study compared PTCAs done from 1977 to 1981 to those done from 1985 to 1986. Overall success rates, where the patient had reduction in narrowing by 20% in all lesions attempted without death, myocardial infarction, or subsequent need for coronary bypass surgery, increased from 61% to 78%. Attempts in which the patient had at least one lesion successfully reduced went from about 69% in the old groups to 91% in the new. The need for emergency bypass surgery following PTCA was also reduced for the new group compared with the old. This was particularly true for those patients with single-vessel disease. An even more significant difference between the two groups was a sharp decrease in elective bypass surgery following PTCA for the new group.

More complex or high-risk cases are now being selected for this form of angioplasty than in its earlier phase. High-risk cases include patients with multiple vessel disease, multiple lesion dilatation, advanced age, prior coronary bypass surgery, poor left ventricular function, and left main coronary artery disease requiring dilation (Hartzler et al., 1988). The National Institute Registry Study showed a significantly higher proportion of the 1985–1986 cases to have multivessel disease, poor left ventricular function, previous myocardial infarction, and previous bypass surgery (Detre et al., 1988).

PTCA is being used fairly extensively for patients with multivessel disease with acceptable outcomes (Cowley et al., 1985). A study by Hartzler and associates of 6,500 procedures done at the Mid-America Heart Institute demonstrates treatment of multiple lesions alone may not increase risk of death for the patient. When they excluded cases with advanced age, poor left ventricular function, prior bypass surgery, and left main coronary artery disease, they found patients undergoing multiple-lesion PTCA had mortality rates equivalent to those who underwent a single lesion procedure (Hartzler et al., 1988).

There have been some comparisons made between PTCA and bypass surgery (Reeder et al., 1984; Morris, 1988; OTA, 1985; Arcidi et al., 1988). PTCA is obviously the less-invasive technique and therefore will result in fewer hospital days and a shorter disability period for the patient. PTCA is substantially lower in cost. However, it is not the best treatment for all patients, and PTCA failure can result in emergency or elective bypass surgery being performed.

On the other hand, there are patients who will not tolerate a surgical procedure but can benefit from PTCA, or whose condition does not warrant the more traumatic bypass procedure. Several studies are underway to compare the role of PTCA with that of coronary artery bypass grafting for the treatment of patients with multivessel disease (Holmes, Reeder & Vlietstra, 1988). Arcidi and associates feel PTCA and bypass surgery should be viewed as complementary treatment modalities rather than competitive modes of therapy (Arcidi et al., 1988).

PTCA's big advantage over bypass surgery in the treatment of patients with coronary artery disease is its substantially lower cost. When PTCA was used originally, case coding resulted in a high-paying surgical DRG that included many more costly procedures. It since has been reclassified into a lower-paying DRG. However, use of PTCA is affected by other economic factors. If its use is unsuccessful and bypass surgery must be performed during the same hospitalization, the hospital is paid the DRG rate for the surgery; the OTA assessment was that this should work to encourage PTCA use.

The number of PTCAs is continuing to increase as providers become more aggressive in using it in treating coronary artery disease. National statistics indicate the number of procedures between 1985 and 1987 grew from 100,000 to an estimated 200,000. As the number of PTCAs increases, the number of bypass surgeries remains high at approximately 250,000 a year (Baim & Ignatius, 1988).

Not surprisingly, the success of the angioplasty procedure has lead to new techniques being developed for the treatment of other heart disease. Percutaneous balloon valvoplasty is used to treat various acquired heart valve stenoses in adults. Children are being treated with catheter procedures to provide nonsurgical correction for some congenital heart diseases (Baim, 1988).

More recently, there has been experimentation and some use of lasers in the revascularization of peripheral and coronary arteries. One method used is a hot-tip metal cap on the end of a catheter. The energy source to heat the cap is supplied by a laser. A less-expensive power source in the form of a radio frequency hot-tip catheter has also been used. The Excimer and other pulsed lasers, because of minimal heat trauma and their precision, show potential for coronary applications (Litvack et al., 1988).

Extracorporeal Shock Wave Lithotripsy (ESWL)

About 5% of the world's population experience the formation of stones in the urinary tract (Miller-Catchpole, 1988a). Sometimes the stone can be passed out of the body spontaneously. In other cases, until the 1950s, only surgical removal of the stone was available as an alternative treatment.

Today, there are several procedures less traumatic than surgery available to deal with urinary tract stones so they can be passed out of the body. These are ESWL and ultrasonic lithotripsy. The latter is the oldest and was first attempted in 1953 (Miller-Catchpole, 1988b). Using this method, ultrasonic energy is transferred to the stone using a rod or probe causing the stone to fracture. It is less invasive than direct surgical removal and, therefore, requires a shorter hospital stay and recuperative period for the patient.

However, the procedure requires the probe to be in direct contact with the stone. The probe must be introduced through a scoping device to allow contact to be made. The process generates heat which is dissipated using an irrigation system. A device similar to a wire basket is used to hold the stone so pressure may be applied with the probe. There is considerable pain associated with this procedure and it must be done under general anesthesia. The use of a new type probe that is able to break up the stone without applying pressure can eliminate the need for the wire basket (Miller-Catchpole, 1988b).

In 1984, the Food and Drug Administration (FDA) approved ESWL, a device that allows lithotripsy to be performed without introducing a probe into the body (OTA, 1985). This technology was developed by Dornier Systems of West Germany in conjunction with C. Chaussy (Kraebber & Torres, 1988). The first clinical trials were conducted in 1980 after about six years of developmental work. Chaussy and associates reported the results of their first 20 cases late in 1980 (Chaussy et al., 1980) and again in 1982 (Chaussy et al., 1982) with the experience of additional cases.

In this procedure the patient is suspended in a tank of degassified and demineralized warm water. A device generates a focused shock wave whose precisely controlled impact point causes the stone to break up. The particles formed, known as gravel, are able, in most cases, to pass spontaneously through the urinary tract (Miller-Catchpole, 1988a; Reilly & Torosian, 1988).

ESWL appears to be the procedure of choice for kidney stones and stones in the proximal (closest to the kidney) end of the ureter. This is particularly true when ureter stones can be moved back into the renal pelvis before pulverization is done. The manipulation of the stone requires the introduction of a scope. Stones lodged in the distal (closest to the bladder) end of the ureter are not as successfully treated by ESWL because most of the delivered energy is absorbed by the bony pelvis. There has been some success with ESWL in treating these stones through the soft-tissue window of the pelvis (Miller-Catchpole, 1988a).

ESWL takes less time to perform than the ultrasound procedure. The latter treatment can take anywhere from one to three hours, while ESWL usually takes less than an hour. If no manipulation of the stone is required, the ESWL procedure can be done with spinal or epidural rather than general anesthesia. Also, the hospital stay is usually several days shorter (Reilly & Torosian, 1988).

A new piezoelectric lithotriptor has been developed that allows ESWL to be done ''dry.'' The patient is positioned in contact with a water-filled cushion in place of being submerged in a tank. Not only does the piezoelectric lithotriptor have the advantage of not requiring immersion and a specific room for it to be used, it was discovered that by reducing the firing rate the stone could be destroyed with no pain to the patient (Vallencian et al., 1988). In many cases this eliminates the need for anesthesia. Some patients are now being treated successfully on an outpatient basis (Marberger et al., 1988; Vallencian et al., 1988). The FDA has approved the Dornier HM4, another type of dry lithotriptor, for use in the United States (Reilly & Torosian, 1988).

Use of ESWL for upper urinary stones is covered under Medicare. Since it is noninvasive, it now gets assigned under available ICD–9–CM procedure codes, not to a surgical DRG, but to the higher-paying of two possible medical DRGs for urinary stone treatment. The same code is used for ultrasonic lithotripsy, but then it is normally used with a code for incision, indicating the minor surgical procedure in which the device is used to fragment the stone before removal. Using both codes results in surgical DRG assignment paying about double the medical DRG amount.

By itself, the PPS might discourage ESWL adoption or its use for Medicare patients. The relationship between the PPS and capital costs and outpatient services are issues here because the major expenditure for the device is its initial capital cost for installation. But Congress decided late in 1987 not to permit folding capital costs into the DRGs at this time, and also cut Medicare capital payments for the next two years (see Mullner, Chap. 15). However, the diffusion of ESWL units into U.S. hospitals has proceeded at a faster rate than orginally anticipated by the developer.

Additionally, there are informal reports that a significant number of ESWL procedures now are being done in combination with a percutaneous procedure. The inference is that the justification for this is medical and not financial. In practice, the basic noninvasive ESWL procedure is not effective in all cases. Hence the change in procedure in some cases. However, those ESWL procedures being done in combination with a percutaneous procedure would be paid at the higher-paying surgical DRG rate in contrast to the medical DRG rate.

The 1985 OTA report mentioned earlier discussed the potential PPS impacts on four other emerging technologies besides PTCA and ESWL. These were intraocular lenses (IOLs); thrombolytic therapy for acute myocardial infarction; therapeutic drug monitoring; and implantable infusion pumps.

IOLs are implanted directly in the eye to replace a natural lens; they have become the preferred method of restoring sight for most patients after cataract surgery. They are an example of a technology recently established as a standard procedure that both raises costs and enhances quality. The improvement in visual acuity relative to contact lenses or glasses is so significant that they have become the treatment of choice. This is among general improvements in the treatment of cataract patients.

While Medicare still will pay for cataract surgery on an inpatient basis under appropriate conditions, this is now tightly controlled by careful PRO scrutiny. This, presumably, has removed the issue of financial incentives for hospitals, physicians, and beneficiaries relative to deciding on inpatient versus outpatient surgery for cataracts. The surgery mostly is being performed on an outpatient basis.

A more recent approach to the treatment of acute myocardial infarction uses thrombolytic agents to dissolve blood clots blocking a coronary artery. The drug can be given intravenously with administration starting immediately at home or in an ambulance, or injected directly into the coronary artery using cardiac catheterization. The latter is a more expensive and involved process. As a result there is great interest in those agents that are effective when administered intravenously.

When the Health Care Financing Administration (HCFA) decided to cover these drugs, there was concern that both methods could be assigned to the same DRG. This would provide an incentive to use the lowest-cost method of administration and the least-costly drug. The use of the therapy could be encouraged if it resulted in assignment to a high-paying DRG. On the other hand, if its use did not result in coding the patient into a higher-paying DRG, the PPS incentive for adoption of the technology would depend on whether it lowered the costs of treating patients. At this point, ProPAC has recommended that the use of these thrombolytic agents not be reflected within any specific DRG, but that there be a general increase in hospital payments under the PPS to account for the cost of treating patients with these drugs. This would be as part of the discretionary adjustment factor in the annual update of DRG prices.

The implantable infusion pump and therapeutic drug monitoring are technological developments that can improve the quality of drug therapy. The implantable infusion pump can eliminate problems connected with the use of external pumps and catheterization systems including, as mentioned earlier, prolonged hospitalization. However, its full cost implications are unclear. There are potential quality advantages, but the implantable pump appears to be more expensive than alternate mechanisms. Also, no single ICD–9–CM procedure code adequately represents the major cost of the pump, its initial surgical implantation, nor is its use tied to any single DRG. It is probable that the cost-minimizing incentives of the PPS will work against routine adoption.

Therapeutic drug monitoring assesses the concentration of a drug in a patient's blood serum. The technology has become accepted practice for a variety of drugs. It has aroused interest because of expected positive effects on the cost and quality of medical care. PPS should encourage this technology to the extent improved testing costs less than the savings it generates. However, if therapeutic drug monitoring improves patient outcomes but increases the overall cost of care, at least in the first stages of diffusion, the effect of the PPS may be to depress its use or discourage its expansion to new drugs.

The relationship to PPS does not appear to have been clarified further since the OTA report for these last two technologies. For both, their applicability is more diffuse than for the others discussed and, as a result, it would be more difficult to tie a PPS policy objective to a specific DRG payment decision. However, the added costs for using either or both could be reflected within the recalibration or updating of DRG prices.

TECHNOLOGY ISSUES: CONCLUDING COMMENTS

Innovations in health care technology in recent years have sparked a revolution in patient care. These have affected the definition of treatable conditions and expected treatment outcomes. Various reimbursement and organization factors interplay with the emergence of new technology. While technology expenditures have increased, they have reduced, in many cases, the need for inpatient care and created the potential for treatment in alternate-care settings.

Health care innovations may or may not hold the promise of being cost reducing for a given episode of hospitalization initially or at any time in the future. Any cost benefit may be for the overall health system or for society as a whole. This would be the case if the major benefit of a new technology rested in a reduced need for future care or in an improved productive capacity of the patient. However, the hospital will risk its own financial situation if its technology decision-making process ignores immediate and potential future cost issues directly affecting the hospital. The general implications of this for future developments in health care and health care technology must be considered.

Cost-cutting pressures combined with new technologies have encouraged more outpatient care, creating an "occupancy crisis" among hospitals. Faced with empty beds, hospitals have reacted by trying to encourage more use of inpatient services in order to generate all-important revenues.

Paradoxically, the very measures that were supposed to encourage cost-cutting have created an incentive for buying more and often high-cost technology. Possessing state-of-the-art medical technology is an important part of the hospital's strategy for attracting patients, or more to the point, attracting area physicians to use the hospital as the facility of choice for their patients. Having the latest advances in technology allows hospitals to project the requisite image of high-quality care and helps in their efforts to keep occupancy rates up.

Pressure to economize comes also from the growth of "managed care" systems. HMOs and PPOs encourage providers to adopt much more careful management of resources. Under this system, hospitals see their customers as the HMO or PPO.

Such group buyers of health care are creating a competitive market for hospitals. They also want quality assessment. This new businesslike atmosphere eventually will produce a more centralized budgeting and decision-making process within health care organizations, in which cost control will play a bigger and bigger role. Marketers of medical technology products will have to deal with this new reality that will produce a reduction in the number of beds available and a new emphasis on sound business procedures.

A complicating factor in the situation is the relationship between technology and the health care system, one that is different from traditional industries. The process technology used in health care delivery can potentially alter the definition of the desired end product, health or wellness. It presents a series of ethical issues. The intent of the care to be provided using technological innovations raises the quantity- versus quality-of-life issue. Consumers fight to have input into decisions that affect their right to die. Physicians and other care providers struggle against taking action that is contrary to what they have been taught to do: sustain life. Policymakers try to establish rules and guidelines that will give order and direction to the decision-making process as well as protect the care givers and consumers.

We can do more than ever before in the treatment of patients, many of whom previously would have died of their conditions. Who we do it to and with what realistically expected outcomes affect issues ranging from cost and use of resources that are not unlimited, to concerns over the potential risks and benefits of treatment. Innovations in technology are never immediately accessible, available, and affordable to all patients who could potentially benefit from their application. Aside from the inevitable time lags in the diffusion of new technology, society rarely devotes sufficient resources to make any care modality universally available.

The ability to do more often increases the risks to the patient. The use of some technology may, because of its invasive nature, result in damage rather than help for the individual. Are the potential benefits worth the potential risks? What are the potential hazards, including legal ones, of not applying certain techniques? What are the social, psychological, and economic costs to the patient, the family, and the larger society of delaying the inevitability of death in certain cases? Advances in health care technology constantly expand the range of situations for which these are relevant questions. When we could do less, fewer decisions had to be made.

5

Assessment of Medical Technologies in Support of Peer Review: Outcomes of In-Hospital Care in 1983–1985

Henry Krakauer

The Bureau of Health Standards and Quality of the Health Care Financing Administration (HCFA) is charged with the assurance of the appropriateness and effectiveness of the medical care provided to patients enrolled in the federal government's Medicare program (Dans, Weiner & Otter, 1985; Rock, 1985; Stern & Epstein, 1985). To assist in the discharge of this responsibility, the bureau has initiated the systematic monitoring of the outcomes—mortality, morbidity, disability, and cost—associated with the delivery of the services supported by the program. The principal objective of this activity is to identify the aspects of medical care that have a significant potential for adverse consequences to the patient. However, the monitoring of secular trends in the utilization and effectiveness of medical care also permits the assessment of the impact of the bureau's activities as well as of the effects of technologic and administrative changes.

Few examples of the use of nationwide data for epidemiologic monitoring and analysis exist. A number of registries that acquire data on specific disease entities such as arthritis (Fries, 1984) and end-stage renal disease (The 21st Congress of the European Dialysis and Transplant Association, 1984) or therapeutic interventions such as bone marrow transplantation (Speck et al., 1984) have been established in the United States and elsewhere. U.S. national data have been used recently to characterize rates of performance and subsequent mortality of selected surgical procedures (Riley & Lubitz, 1985), readmission rates (Anderson & Steinberg, 1984), the management of patients with end-stage renal disease (Eggers, Connorton & McMullan, 1984; Eggers, 1984; Krakauer et al., 1983), and to conduct an in-depth assessment of a new therapeutic agent used in organ transplantation (Krakauer, 1986), demonstrating the utility of such data in medical and in administrative/policy applications.

Although the National Center for Health Statistics (NCHS) compiles voluminous data on the health status of the U.S. population (Golden, Wilson & Kavet, 1984), extensive information on the continuum of care is collected principally by HCFA, albeit only for persons eligible for coverage under Medicare, about 90% of whom are over 65.

The analyses presented below characterize the outcomes achieved overall with inpatient care in short-stay hospitals for patients discharged in the calendar years 1983–1985. More detailed is the analysis of outcomes of nine tracer conditions, four medical and five surgical, for which more adequate diagnostic data began to be entered on the billing forms in 1984 in conjunction with the implementation of the Prospective Payment System (PPS) (Health Care Financing Administration, 1983).

The overall focus of this volume is on the relationships between health care, technology, and the economic environment for care delivery, i.e., the changes in the Medicare reimbursement approach and the increasingly competitive marketplace. The assessment reviewed in this chapter permits consideration as to whether implementing the Medicare changes has had a negative impact on the outcomes of inpatient care. If there is an indication of adverse effect, this may suggest a possible relationship to Medicare-based changes within hospitals in patient care practices, use of technology, and other factors. Alternatively, if there is no evidence of adverse effect, it would suggest that whatever changes have been instituted within hospitals under Medicare have not been detrimental to patient welfare.

MATERIALS AND METHODS

The data sets assembled by HCFA and used in the present analyses are based on bills submitted for hospitalization, for ambulatory care, and for limited intermediate care and noncustodial skilled nursing facility services. In addition, certain information pertaining to the patients, such as status of eligibility and date of death, are obtained from the Social Security Administration (SSA). The databases are subjected to electronic checks for internal consistency and for whether values fell within acceptable ranges, but they were not otherwise verified. For the analyses presented below, a 5% sample of patients who were admitted to and discharged from short-stay hospitals in 1983–1985 was selected on the basis of the last two digits of their Social Security numbers. The sample is, therefore, for practical purposes, a random sample. In addition, because computational resources at HCFA are rather limited, a further 20% subsample (every fifth case) was used for the life-table and proportional hazards modeling analyses of the overall populations. Because of the absence of adequate diagnostic data until the last quarter of 1983, assignment of patients to the tracer conditions could not be made for admissions that occurred prior to that time, and analysis of the tracer conditions is limited to 1984 and 1985. The full 5% sample was used in all analyses pertaining to the tracer conditions.

The direct comparisons of 1984 and 1985 hospitalizations (see Tables 5.1–5.5) were performed on data received by HCFA and SSA within 18 months of the end of the year evaluated, i.e., by June 1986 for 1984 and June 1987 for 1985. All other analyses were performed on data received by June 1986.

To permit more detailed analysis of diagnostically relatively homogeneous groups, "tracer" conditions were identified by means of diagnosis-related groups (DRGs) and consisted of: (1) heart failure and shock (DRG 127), (2) acute myocardial infarction (DRGs 121–123), (3) pneumonia (DRGs 89–90), (4) gastrointestinal hemorrhage (DRGs 174–175), (5) cholecystectomy (DRGs 195–198), (6) major joint procedures (DRG 209), (7) transurethral prostatectomy (DRGs 336–337 and the transurethral procedures [ICD–9–CM codes 60.2 and 57.49] in DRGs 306–307), (8) coronary artery bypass graft surgery (DRGs 106–107), and (9) permanent cardiac pacemaker implants (DRGs 115–116).

The impact of case-mix on mortality rates of the aggregate populations was estimated by means of "major" conditions selected on clinical and empiric grounds as likely to be associated with a distinctly high or a distinctly low probability of death subsequent to hospitalization. These major conditions were identified by the ICD–9–CM codes of the principal diagnoses given in the Appendix and consisted of, in the high-risk group, (1) malignancy, (2) severe acute heart disease, (3) severe chronic heart disease, (4) cerebrovascular accidents, (5) sepsis, (6) severe trauma, (7) pulmonary disease, (8) renal disease, (9) gastroenterologic catastrophes, and (10) metabolic and electrolyte disturbances; in the low-risk group, of (11) low-risk heart disease, (12) gastrointestinal disease, (13) genitourinary disease, (14) gynecologic disease, (15) ophthalmologic disease, and (16) orthopedic conditions. These diagnostic categories include about 70% of patients and 80% of deaths subsequent to hospitalization.

The impact of the complexity of the patients' condition within the tracer conditions was explored by means of a specification of coexisting, principally chronic, conditions (comorbidities) coded as secondary diagnoses on the bill for the index admission. Up to four of these were available. The comorbidities were identified by their ICD–9–CM codes, also given in the Appendix, and included (1) malignancy, (2) ischemic heart disease and failure, (3) chronic pulmonary disease, (4) chronic renal disease, (5) chronic liver disease (571–572), (6) degenerative cerebral disease and psychosis, (7) hypertensive disease, (8) diabetes, and (9) autoimmune disease. They were selected on the basis of the belief that their presence would complicate the management of the patient and increase the probability of an adverse outcome.

For the purpose of survival analysis, time at risk was computed from the first day of the first hospital admission of the patient. The patient was followed until death or 30 days beyond the end of the last calendar year in the period of observation, at which time he or she was withdrawn alive from study (censored).

Cumulative mortality rates subsequent to hospitalization were computed by the actuarial or life-table method.

The Cox proportional hazards model (Cox & Oakes, 1984; Harrell, 1983), was used to identify covariates (factors) significantly associated with mortality and to gain an impression as to their relative importance. These factors included demographic characteristics of the patients: age; sex; race (black/not black; other than white or black); case-mix in the form of major conditions in the analyses of the aggregate populations; and comorbidities in the case of the analyses of the tracer conditions. In addition, the relative risk of death associated with hospitalization in 1985 rather than 1984 was estimated by treating an indicator of such an admission as a covariate. The purpose of this computation was the assessment of the impact of the major administrative changes phased in during 1984, the Prospective Payment System (PPS) and the peer review organizations (PRO). To assure comparability and a fair assessment of the secular trend, the population samples were constructed and survival times were computed separately for each of the two calendar years; only then were the populations combined.

The pattern of morbidity was assessed by means of an analysis of readmissions. In the case on the tracer conditions, the total frequency and the frequency of readmission classified according to cause were calculated from the index admission onward and during specific periods following initial discharge (up to 30 days, 31–180 days, and 181–360 days). For the latter, only those index admissions were used that allowed sufficient follow-up to cover the period of observation. Thus, for readmissions in the period 181–360 days following discharge, only those index admissions were used that resulted in a discharge at least 360 days prior to the end of 1985 and from which the patient had survived at least 180 days. The causes for readmission were identified by means of DRGs: pulmonary (DRGs 79–102); cardiovascular (DRGs 103–145); gastrointestinal (DRGs 146–208); musculoskeletal (DRGs 209–256); genitourinary (DRGs 302–352); and complications of treatment (DRGs 452–453). The time to first readmission was also analyzed both for readmissions for all causes and for readmissions for related causes, defined as those involving the same organ system as the initial admission, except in the cases of heart failure and shock and of pneumonia where both pulmonary and cardiovascular causes were taken to be related to the initial admission. The period of observation was from the day after the day of discharge to the end of 1985, and persons who died without having been readmitted were withdrawn at the time of death. As in the case of the analysis of mortality rates, the actuarial method and the Cox proportional hazards model were used to assess time to first readmission.

The cost of ambulatory care was used as a surrogate measure of morbidity not requiring hospitalization. Similarly, the only measures of disability available in the HCFA billing data are the charges for Home Health Agency and Medicare-covered skilled nursing facility services, given herein as charges for "supportive care."

Multiple linear regression techniques were used to compute the contributions of the previously defined potentially predictive factors to overall charges accumulated from the admission onward.

The charges for medical care analyzed for 1984 and 1985 consist of all billed charges for services provided by hospitals, both inpatient and outpatient, but only those charges for physician services and ambulatory care not furnished by hospitals deemed "reasonable" by the insurance carriers who serve as agents of HCFA.

RESULTS

The demographic characteristics of patients hospitalized in 1983–1985 and the incidence of high-risk conditions on initial admission in 1984 and 1985 are shown in Table 5.1. The number hospitalized in both years is undoubtedly understated because of delays in receipt and processing of bills. However, as equal amounts of time elapsed for the accumulation of the bills (18 months from the end of the calendar year) in both years, they may be compared fairly. Overall, there is a continuing downward trend in the number of patients receiving hospital care and of the duration of their stays, and a continuing trend upward in the proportion in the most-aged group. There is also an increase in the proportion of conditions associated with a higher risk of death and a decrease in the proportion of conditions associated with a lower risk of death (see Table 5.1).

The lower frequency of index admissions is not accompanied by an increase in readmissions (see Table 5.2). The proportion of patients with multiple admissions in 1985 ise understated because delays in the processing of bills affects most severely those generated later in the year. Nevertheless, a deterioration in the effectiveness of inpatient care, which should have resulted in a higher incidence of readmission, is not evident from these data. The same inference may be drawn from the population-based mortality rates (the total number of deaths among Medicare beneficiaries in a calendar year divided by the number of beneficiaries enrolled at mid year) given in Table 5.3.

On the other hand, there is a distinct increase in the cumulative mortality of patients following an initial hospitalization in 1985 compared to 1984 or 1983 (see Table 5.4). The higher mortality rate is clearly evident in the first interval, i.e., within 30 days of admission, and it appears to increase thereafter. The extent to which this divergence can be accounted for by changes in demographic composition and case mix is explored in Table 5.5. The relative risk is the ratio of the probabilities of dying per unit time of two populations differing in the risk factor specified, but with equal relative frequencies of all the other risk factors (covariates) used in the model. Thus, women have less than three-quarters the change of dying subsequent to hospitalization than men of equivalent age, racial composition, and incidence of the major conditions analyzed. The high-risk conditions, with the exception of trauma, are indeed highly predictive of

Table 5.1
Patient Characteristics: First Admissions in the Calendar Year

	1983	1984	1985
Total	7.3 million	6.8 million	6.0 million
Age:			
0-64	10.6%	10.0%	10.0%
65-69	22.2	21.9	21.1
70-74	21.8	21.5	21.6
75-79	18.8	19.2	19.1
80-84	14.0	14.4	14.4
85 +	12.7	13.1	13.8
Sex:			
Male	43.8	43.8	44.1
Female	56.2	56.2	55.9
Race:			
White	88.6	88.2	88.0
Black	7.8	8.1	8.2
Other	3.6	3.7	3.8
Major Conditions:[1]			
High Risk--			
Malignancy		7.0%	7.3%
Severe Acute Heart Disease		3.5	3.9
Severe Chronic Heart Disease		4.6	4.9
Cerebrovascular Accidents		3.2	3.7
Sepsis		0.4	0.6
Severe Trauma		2.4	2.8
Pulmonary Disease		7.4	8.0
Renal Disease		0.8	0.8
Gastroenterologic Catastrophes		1.8	1.9
Metabolic and Electrolyte Disorders		1.5	1.9
Low Risk--			
Gastrointestinal Disease		10.4	9.9
Genitourinary		4.4	4.5
Gynecologic Disease		1.0	1.0
Orthopedic Disorders		7.1	7.1
Ophthalmologic Disease		5.4	2.4
Low-Risk Heart Disease		8.8	9.2
Average Length of stay:	9.2 days	8.4 days	8.1 days

Note: 1. The ICD-9-CM codes that define these conditions are
         given in the Appendix.

death. However, they are somewhat less so in 1985 than in 1984, indicating that
the reference group of the hospitalized population was also more severely ill in
the latter year. If both the demographic characteristics and the measure of case
mix used here are taken into account, the excess risk of admission in 1985
compared to 1984 is nearly entirely accounted for. Taken in conjunction with

Table 5.2
Readmissions

Number of Readmissions	Proportion of Persons[1]		
	1983	1984	1985
None	65.0%	65.8%	66.3%
One	21.3	20.9	20.6
Two	7.9	7.7	7.5
Three	3.2	3.0	3.1
Four and more	2.7	2.6	2.6

Note: 1. Proportion of persons readmitted in the calendar year specified following an index admission in that year.

Table 5.3
Population-Based Mortality Rates for Calendar Year

	1983	1984	1985
Medicare enrollees (in millions)	30.03	30.46	31.08
Raw mortality rate	5.08%	5.08%	5.10%
Age-adjusted mortality rate (ref. year: 1983)	(5.07%)	5.05%	5.06%

the fact that the age-adjusted population-based mortality rate is not different in the two years, the increase in postadmission mortality rates appears to have been due to a greater preponderance of ominous diagnoses. As deaths subsequent to hospitalization in 1984 and 1985 account for about 64% of all deaths of Medicare beneficiaries in those years, it is unlikely that an increase in postadmission mortality rates of the magnitude observed, had it been due to a deterioration of the effectiveness of care, would have failed to have been reflected in the population-based mortality rate.

A more detailed analysis of the outcomes of hospital care is presented for nine tracer conditions identified principally by a panel of physicians representing the PROs as being of particular interest because of potential problems in the patterns of case selection and management. The characteristics of the patients hospitalized

Table 5.4
Cumulative Mortality Rates: First Admissions in the Calendar Year

Days after admission	1983	1984	1985
30	5.7±0.1%	5.9±0.1%	6.6±0.1%
90	9.8±0.1	10.2±0.1	11.1±0.2
180	13.5±0.1	13.8±0.2	15.2±0.2
270	16.2±0.2	16.8±0.2	18.2±0.2
360	19.1±0.2	19.7±0.2	21.2±0.2

for four medical conditions and five surgical procedures and their patterns of mortality are summarized in Table 5.6 and their patterns of morbidity requiring hospitalization in Table 5.7. The cases investigated in these tables are the first recorded admissions for the conditions or procedures specified in the period 1984–1985. Tables 5.8 and 5.9 present similar analyses separately for 1984 and 1985 to examine secular trends in outcomes more exhaustively. It must be noted that the data in Tables 5.6 and 5.7 are not simple averages of the data in Tables 5.8 and 5.9 because the former exclude patients readmitted in 1985 for conditions for which they had been admitted in 1984, but the latter, to assure symmetry in the relation of these two years with 1983–1984 in terms of readmissions, do not.

The differing patterns of mortality consequent to hospitalization for the tracer conditions clearly demonstrate the differences of the underlying status of the health of the patient. The medical admissions and the implantation of a cardiac pacemaker are precipitated by organ failure. They are, therefore, characterized by both a high initial mortality as well as a persistent elevation in probability of dying per unit time. The criteria for selection of patients for coronary artery bypass surgery appear to exclude effectively those with compromised cardiac function. Hence, although the procedure itself entails a rather high risk in the Medicare population with a postoperative mortality rate of 5.5% within 30 days of admission, those who do survive the operation have a good prognosis, only an additional 8% or so dying in the subsequent 23 months.

Among the comorbidities, malignancy, chronic renal disease, and chronic liver disease appear to be consistently and substantially adverse prognostic factors (see Tables 5.6, 5.8, and 5.9). Diabetes and chronic cardiac disease (ischemic heart disease and failure) are also uniformly adverse, but with a limited magnitude of impact. Degenerative cerebral disease and chronic psychosis appear important only in three of the surgical procedures with intrinsically low mortality rates, i.e., where the absolute effect on the mortality rate is quite small. Most interestingly, hypertensive disease appears in all cases to be a favorable prognostic factor. However, it must be noted that this is so after differences in the incidence

Table 5.5
Mortality Risk Factors (Cox Proportional Hazards Model)

	1983	1984	1985
		RELATIVE RISKS[1]	
Sex (female vs. male)	(0.67)	0.76(0.65)	0.76(0.69)
Race (black vs. others)	(1.21)	1.08(1.25)	1.08(1.17)
Age (80 vs. 65 yrs)	(1.98)	2.00(2.09)	2.03(2.03)
Length of Stay (+7 days)	(1.11)	-- (1.09)	-- (1.10)
Major Conditions[2]:			
High Risk--			
Malignancy		3.82	3.18
Severe Acute Heart Disease		4.24	3.82
Severe Chronic Heart Disease		2.60	2.55
Cerebrovascular Accidents		3.17	2.86
Sepsis		3.92	3.15
Severe Trauma		1.37	1.12
Pulmonary Disease		1.98	1.95
Renal Disease		3.17	2.56
Gastroenterologic Catastrophes		1.94	1.80
Metabolic and Electrolyte Disorders		2.28	2.08
Low Risk--			
Gastrointestinal Disease		0.76	0.77
Genitourinary Disease		0.72	0.70
Gynecologic Disease		0.21	0.27
Orthopedic Disorders		0.48	0.43
Ophthalmologic Disease		0.23	0.28
Low-Risk Heart Disease		0.85	0.77
1985 vs. 1984 admissions		1.09 (P <.0001)	
1985 vs. 1984 admissions, allowing for differences in demographic mix		1.07 (P <.0001)	
1985 vs. 1984 admissions, allowing for differences in demographic mix and "Major Conditions"		1.02 (P >.0.25)	

Notes:
1. Relative risks in parentheses were computed without inclusion of "Major Conditions".

2. The ICD-9-CM codes that define these conditions are given in the Appendix.

of chronic diseases that can be precipitated by hypertension—chronic cardiac, cerebral, and renal disease—have been compensated for. In addition, it must be noted that only four additional diagnoses are reported on the bills. It may, therefore, be that hypertensive disease is entered only if other, more serious comorbidities are not present and complications did not occur. Hence the coding of hypertensive disease as a comorbidity may be a marker of wellness rather than illness. This phenomenon has been observed in other low-risk additional

Table 5.6
Admissions during Calendar Years 1984 and 1985: Outcomes of Care for Nine Selected Conditions or Procedures

	HFS[1]	AMI	PNU	GIH	CSX	JTP	TUP	CAB	PCM
Percent of all patients hospitalized	6.73%	5.22%	5.61%	2.58%	2.09%	2.66%	3.64%	1.16%	1.09
Patient Characteristics									
Age: Under 65	6.5%	7.5%	7.4%	7.3%	8.8%	5.4%	3.7%	12.9%	3.2%
65-74	32.0	44.9	33.4	36.4	54.7	40.1	52.0	71.8	32.1
75-84	39.5	35.6	36.1	36.8	29.5	38.8	36.2	15.0	44.1
84 and over	22.1	12.0	23.0	19.4	7.0	15.6	8.0	0.4	20.6
Sex: Male	43.0%	46.9%	48.2%	45.2%	39.0%	28.6%	--	69.6%	47.2%
Race: White	86.7%	90.4%	89.6%	87.9%	90.8%	92.5%	89.3%	94.1%	91.0%
Black	9.7	5.9	7.0	8.4	4.4	4.1	6.7	2.3	6.0
Comorbidities[2]									
Malignancy	3.2%	1.4%	6.1%	4.9%	3.2%	1.8%	7.0%	0.7%	1.6%
Autoimmune Disease	0.9	0.6	1.3	1.7	0.7	2.0	0.3	0.4	0.4
Chronic Liver Disease	0.7	0.2	0.5	2.8	2.9	0.3	0.1	0	0.2
Chronic Renal Disease	4.7	2.1	2.2	2.6	0.6	0.6	1.0	0.9	1.6
Degenerative Cerebral Disease & Psychosis	1.6	1.1	3.3	2.2	0.8	2.2	0.8	0.3	1.2
Hypertensive Disease	13.4	16.2	9.5	11.9	5.1	17.5	10.7	17.5	17.4
Ischemic Heart Disease & Failure	--	--	35.2	23.6	21.0	18.7	17.6	--	--
Diabetes	8.2	7.6	4.8	3.9	4.6	2.3	2.6	5.0	4.2
Chronic Pulmonary Disease	15.8	8.6	25.5	8.0	6.5	5.6	8.5	6.0	5.3
Pattern of Mortality									
Cumulative Mortality									
Days After Admission									
30	13.3%	25.3%	13.8%	7.8%	2.5%	2.7%	1.1%	5.5%	3.4%
90	22.3	30.5	20.8	13.0	42.8	5.3	3.0	7.5	7.3
180	29.4	34.4	26.1	17.4	6.6	7.7	5.4	9.0	11.8
270	35.2	37.1	29.9	20.8	8.2	9.2	7.5	9.9	14.8
360	40.1	39.5	33.2	24.0	9.7	10.6	9.6	10.7	17.4
540	47.5	43.6	38.7	28.7	11.9	13.2	13.6	11.8	22.4
630	50.9	45.3	41.0	31.1	12.9	14.4	15.7	12.6	25.2
720	54.2	47.1	43.5	33.4	13.8	15.4	17.4	13.4	28.6

	HFS	AMI	PNU	GIH	CSX	JTP	TUP	CAB	PCM
Relative Risk of Dying[3]									
Female vs. Male	0.76	0.96	0.72	0.87	0.74	0.72	--	1.15	0.76
Black vs. Other Races	0.86	0.92	1.16	(1.10)	1.40	1.36	1.32	1.43	(1.17)
Age, 80 vs. 65	1.47	1.83	1.86	1.88	2.72	3.99	2.70	1.78	1.72
Malignancy	2.25	1.58	3.05	5.00	6.93	4.30	3.19	(1.55)	2.01
Autoimmune Disease	1.22	0.78	(1.06)	(1.00)	(1.38)	(1.33)	1.79	(0.90)	(1.39)
Chronic Liver Disease	1.31	1.85	1.90	3.13	2.94	3.38	(1.10)	--	(1.47)
Chronic Renal Disease	2.08	2.15	2.56	3.25	5.95	5.20	2.20	4.22	2.30
Degenerativae Cerebral Disease & Psychosis	1.15	0.82	1.31	1.51	2.28	1.89	2.00	--	1.24
Hypertensive Disease	0.73	0.63	0.59	0.62	0.69	0.69	0.87	0.55	0.75
Ischemic Heart Disease & Failure	--	--	1.25	1.45	1.41	1.75	1.38	--	--
Diabetes	1.13	1.24	1.20	1.33	1.65	1.91	1.46	(1.05)	(1.53)
Chronic Pulmonary Disease	(0.99)	(0.98)	0.90	1.32	1.41	1.65	1.61	(1.16)	1.29

Note:

1. HFS = congestive heart failure and shock
   AMI = acute myocardial infarction
   PNU = pneumonia
   GIH = gastrointestinal hemorrhage
   CSX = cholecystectomy
   JTP = major joint procedures
   TUP = transurethral prostatectomy
   CAB = coronary artery bypass graft surgery
   PCM = cardiac pacemaker implant

2. Percent of patients within the diagnostic categories with the conditions specified as secondary diagnoses, as defined by the ICD-9-CM codes on the hospital bill.

3. Relative risks were computed by means of the Cox proportional hazards model. The relative risk associated with a comorbidity is the ratio of the probability of dying for patients with that condition to that for demographically similar patients without the condition. Relative risks in parentheses differed from 1.00 with a probability less than 90% (P > 0.1).

Table 5.7
Pattern of Morbidity for Patients Hospitalized in 1984–1985

	HFS	AMI	PNU	GIH	CSX	JTP	TUP	CAB	PCM
PERCENTAGE OF PERSONS AT RISK WITH SPECIFIED NUMBERS OF READMISSIONS									
None	39.9	44.9	51.9	54.1	70.3	64.6	64.3	61.0	53.4
One	26.8	27.9	24.5	23.8	17.6	22.8	20.9	23.0	24.0
Two	14.6	13.4	11.4	10.6	6.5	7.5	7.8	8.6	11.9
Over two	18.7	13.8	12.2	11.5	5.6	5.1	6.9	7.4	10.7
READMISSIONS FOR CAUSES SPECIFIED PER 100 PERSONS AT RISK									
Pulmonary	16.4	8.2	32.3	8.8	4.9	4.6	6.2	5.2	7.3
Cardiovascular	71.6	72.0	20.3	16.8	11.2	8.2	12.1	31.7	44.1
Gastrointestinal	11.8	8.2	10.4	32.7	13.6	6.3	8.3	8.6	9.4
Musculoskeletal	4.5	2.8	5.2	6.1	3.6	17.4	3.5	2.8	3.8
Genitourinary	6.6	4.2	5.6	5.3	3.7	3.1	16.2	3.8	4.4
Complications of Treatment					0.3	0.9	1.9	0.5	0.6
TIME TO FIRST READMISSION									
Cumulative Proportion of Persons Readmitted (All Causes). Days After Initial Discharge									
30	20.3%	20.5%	14.8%	13.7%	7.9%	8.5%	9.6%	14.4%	15.1%
90	38.3	34.5	27.9	26.4	14.7	17.1	18.4	23.9	26.6
180	51.9	44.5	38.7	36.4	21.2	25.3	26.7	31.4	36.4
360	67.1	56.6	52.4	49.4	31.6	36.6	37.8	41.2	50.3
540	74.5	63.7	60.7	58.0	38.3	44.4	45.8	48.0	58.5
720	79.0	69.2	65.8	62.9	44.4	50.5	51.2	51.3	62.8
Relative Risk of Readmission[2]									
Female vs. Male	0.95	(1.00)	0.87	(0.97)	0.85	0.90	--	1.22	(1.02)
Black vs. Other Races	0.94	0.84	(1.02)	(1.05)	1.18	1.13	1.12	(1.18)	1.33
Age, 80 vs. 65	0.95	(0.98)	1.05	1.04	1.19	1.10	1.31	(1.07)	1.11
Malignancy	1.36	1.45	1.82	2.38	2.67	1.74	1.77	1.51	1.58
Chronic Liver Disease	(0.99)	(0.80)	1.24	1.96	1.50	2.43	(1.05)	--	(0.79)
Chronic Renal Disease	1.53	1.65	1.82	2.10	2.82	2.46	1.44	2.21	1.47
Degenerative Cerebral Disease & Psychosis	(0.98)	(0.94)	(1.09)	(1.12)	1.48	(1.17)	1.37	2.14	(0.76)
Hypertensive Disease	0.93	0.92	0.85	0.92	0.86	0.91	0.94	0.83	0.89
Ischemic Heart Disease & Failure	--	--	1.17	1.17	1.28	1.25	1.20	--	-
Diabetes	1.22	1.20	1.29	1.40	1.51	1.48	1.29	1.42	1.22
Chronic Pulmonary Disease	1.07	1.15	1.11	1.31	1.47	1.27	1.28	1.51	(1.13)

Cumulative Proportion of Persons Readmitted (Related Causes[3].)

Days After Initial Discharge

	HFS	AMI	PNU	GIH	CSX	JTP	TUP	CAB	PCM
30	13.5%	15.5%	8.8%	6.1%	2.6%	2.3%	3.2%	7.3%	8.2%
90	26.9	26.5	16.9	11.3	5.0	5.4	6.4	12.6	15.1
180	37.8	33.5	23.7	15.8	7.2	9.1	9.4	17.1	21.2
360	51.5	41.7	34.0	22.8	10.8	14.3	13.1	22.4	29.9
540	59.0	47.3	40.6	27.3	13.5	18.0	16.0	26.1	35.2
720	63.2	51.6	44.9	30.8	15.1	20.2	17.9	29.2	39.6

PRIOR ADMISSIONS

PERCENTAGE OF PERSONS AT RISK WITH SPECIFIED NUMBERS OF PRIOR ADMISSIONS

	HFS	AMI	PNU	GIH	CSX	JTP	TUP	CAB	PCM
None	54.4	67.2	58.3	58.2	62.6	69.8	70.4	30.4	55.1
One	24.1	19.1	21.6	22.1	23.9	19.7	19.5	39.2	25.7
Two	11.0	7.4	9.9	10.1	7.9	6.5	6.2	18.3	10.7
Over two	10.5	6.3	10.2	9.5	5.6	4.1	3.9	12.1	8.5

PRIOR ADMISSIONS FOR CAUSES SPECIFIED PER 100 PERSONS AT RISK

	HFS	AMI	PNU	GIH	CSX	JTP	TUP	CAB	PCM
Pulmonary	13.8	5.8	14.7	8.2	4.1	3.7	4.4	3.1	5.1
Cardiovascular	28.7	23.5	17.6	16.5	12.6	7.0	10.2	98.6	41.1
Gastrointestinal	9.9	7.1	10.6	15.9	23.0	6.5	7.3	5.4	7.1
Musculoskeletal	5.3	3.5	6.8	7.7	3.8	13.8	3.0	2.5	3.9
Genitourinary	5.5	3.7	5.8	5.8	3.3	2.7	10.1	3.3	4.2
Complications of Treatment									

RESOURCES USED IN PRIOR ADMISSIONS PER PERSON ADMITTED

	HFS	AMI	PNU	GIH	CSX	JTP	TUP	CAB	PCM
Length of Stay	18.7[4]	15.1	20.1	19.2	12.0	13.9	12.4	10.6	13.5
	12.4[5]	9.5	12.5	11.8	7.6	8.3	7.6	6.8	8.7
Charges	$10300[4]	7900	9900	9600	6400	6500	7000	7200	7500
	$6200[5]	4800	5800	5600	3800	3900	4000	4900	4700

READMISSIONS WITHIN 30 DAYS

PERCENTAGE OF PERSONS AT RISK WITH SPECIFIED NUMBERS OF READMISSIONS

	HFS	AMI	PNU	GIH	CSX	JTP	TUP	CAB	PCM
None	77.8	72.9	83.6	84.2	91.4	87.9	89.6	83.4	83.6
One	19.3	22.8	14.7	13.9	7.9	11.0	9.4	15.1	14.3
Two	2.6	3.8	1.6	1.8	0.7	0.9	0.9	1.4	1.8
Over two	0.3	0.5	0.2	0.2	0.1	0.2	0.1	0.2	0.2

53

Table 5.7 (continued)

	HFS	AMI	PNU	GIH	CSX	JTP	TUP	CAB	PCM
READMISSIONS FOR CAUSES SPECIFIED PER 100 PERSONS AT RISK									
Pulmonary	2.7	1.5	7.4	1.2	0.7	0.9	0.7	1.8	1.4
Cardiovascular	13.8	24.9	3.3	2.5	1.6	1.5	1.4	8.1	9.8
Gastrointestinal	2.0	1.2	1.6	8.1	3.0	1.1	1.1	1.6	1.5
Musculoskeletal	0.6	0.3	0.6	0.8	0.3	4.7	0.2	0.3	0.4
Genitourinary	1.4	0.6	1.0	1.0	0.7	0.7	3.6	0.6	0.8
Complications of Treatment	0.0	0.0	0.0	0.1	0.2	0.4	1.7	0.3	0.2
RESOURCES USED IN READMISSIONS PER PERSON READMITTED									
Length of Stay	10.8[4]	10.6	11.0	11.0	10.3	14.3	8.7	10.0	9.1
	7.9[5]	7.5	8.0	7.8	7.1	10.2	6.0	7.0	6.7
Charges	$6800[4]	9400	6300	6800	5900	6300	4800	6200	5700
	$4200[5]	5400	3900	4100	3400	4200	2800	3900	3700

READMISSIONS AT 31-180 DAYS

	HFS	AMI	PNU	GIH	CSX	JTP	TUP	CAB	PCM
PERCENTAGE OF PERSONS AT RISK WITH SPECIFIED NUMBERS OF READMISSIONS									
None	53.5	62.2	67.1	67.5	81.5	77.8	76.8	74.5	67.7
One	28.8	24.4	21.9	21.4	13.2	17.3	17.0	18.6	22.5
Two	11.3	8.7	7.2	6.9	3.8	3.8	4.3	4.9	6.5
Over two	6.4	4.7	3.9	4.2	1.5	1.2	2.0	2.0	3.2
READMISSIONS FOR CAUSES SPECIFIED PER 100 PERSONS AT RISK									
Pulmonary	8.6	4.6	15.6	4.9	2.3	2.5	3.3	2.5	3.7
Cardiovascular	38.4	36.5	10.0	8.5	5.4	4.3	6.0	16.6	22.5
Gastrointestinal	6.0	4.6	5.2	16.9	7.0	2.8	4.2	4.6	4.8
Musculoskeletal	2.3	1.3	2.8	3.2	1.8	8.9	1.6	1.5	1.7
Genitourinary	3.3	2.3	2.9	2.8	1.7	1.6	8.7	1.9	2.1
RESOURCES USED IN READMISSIONS PER PERSON READMITTED									
Length of Stay	14.3[4]	12.2	13.4	13.7	11.7	12.8	11.2	10.3	12.0
	9.8[5]	8.1	9.3	9.3	7.7	8.9	7.3	6.9	8.0
Charges	$8500[4]	8700	7500	8300	6700	7400	6700	7100	7200
	$5100[5]	5100	4700	4900	4000	4800	4100	4300	4400

READMISSIONS WITHIN 181-360 DAYS

	HFS	AMI	PNU	GIH	CSX	JTP	TUP	CAB	PCM
PERCENTAGE OF PERSONS AT RISK WITH SPECIFIED NUMBERS OF READMISSIONS									
None	49.4	64.3	59.5	64.8	78.9	76.9	75.9	76.0	66.0
One	30.7	23.7	27.0	23.5	14.9	17.9	17.2	17.1	24.2
Two	12.3	8.0	8.5	7.2	4.3	4.1	4.6	3.9	6.5
Over two	7.6	4.1	5.0	4.5	1.9	1.1	2.4	2.1	3.4
READMISSIONS FOR CAUSES SPECIFIED PER 100 PERSONS AT RISK									
Pulmonary	10.4	4.9	18.7	5.6	2.9	2.3	3.7	2.3	3.8
Cardiovascular	41.1	28.5	13.4	10.4	6.5	4.3	7.2	14.2	22.6
Gastrointestinal	7.5	4.9	6.6	16.6	6.9	3.9	4.8	4.5	5.4
Musculoskeletal	2.9	2.0	3.5	3.6	2.4	8.7	2.2	1.7	2.4
Genitourinary	3.9	2.5	3.5	3.0	1.9	1.6	7.7	2.3	2.3
RESOURCES USED IN READMISSIONS PER PERSON READMITTED									
Length of Stay	14.0[4]	11.8	12.9	12.9	11.3	12.2	11.4	8.8	11.4
	9.6[5]	9.6	8.8	8.5	7.6	8.5	7.5	5.9	7.5
Charges	$8300[4]	4700	7500	7600	6400	7400	6900	5900	6600
	$5100[5]	4700	4600	4500	3800	4700	4300	3700	4200

Notes:

1. The conditions specified are identified in Table 5.6

2. Relative risks were computed by means of the Cox proportional hazards model. Relative risks in parentheses differed from 1.00 with a probability less than 90% (P > 0.1).

3. A cause for readmission was taken to be related to the cause of the initial admission if it involved the same organ system, except that readmissions for disease involving either the pulmonary or cardiovascular systems were taken to be related to initial admissions for heart failure and shock and for pneumonia.

4. Arithmetic means.

5. Geometric means.

Table 5.8
Admissions during Calendar Year 1984: Outcomes of Care for Nine Selected Conditions or Procedures

	HFS	AMI	PNU	GIH	CSX	JTP	TUP	CAB	PCM
Percent of all patients hospitalized[1]	5.93%	4.31%	4.45%	2.13%	1.68%	2.08%	2.95%	0.89%	0.89%
Patient Characteristics									
Age: Under 65	6.7%	7.9%	7.7%	7.4%	8.9%	5.6%	3.8%	12.8%	2.9%
65-74	31.3	44.9	33.4	36.3	54.7	40.1	52.0	73.0	32.6
75-84	40.1	35.3	36.1	36.8	29.3	39.2	36.3	13.9	44.1
84 and over	21.9	11.8	22.8	19.5	7.1	15.2	7.7	0.4	20.4
Sex: Male	43.3%	47.1%	48.7%	46.0%	37.9%	28.1%	--	68.8%	43%
Race: White	86.5%	91.1%	89.7%	87.7%	91.3%	92.4%	89.2%	94.4%	91.0%
Black	9.9	5.5	6.9	8.6	4.4	4.3	6.9	2.2	6.0
Comorbidities[2]									
Malignancy	2.8%	1.4%	5.5%	4.5%	2.9%	1.7%	6.7%	0.6%	1.6%
Autoimmune Disease	0.8	0.6	1.3	1.6	0.7	2.0	0.3	0.3	0.5
Chronic Liver Disease	0.7	0.1	0.5	2.6	2.9	0.3	0.1	0	0.2
Chronic Renal Disease	4.5	1.9	2.1	2.3	0.6	0.5	0.9	0.7	1.5
Degenerative Cerebral Disease & Psychosis	1.5	0.9	3.0	2.0	0.8	2.2	0.8	0.3	0.9
Hypertensive Disease	12.3	15.0	9.1	10.9	14.3	16.7	10.1	16.0	16.7
Ischemic Heart Disease & Failure	--	--	33.8	21.9	20.1	17.8	16.9	--	--
Diabetes	7.6	6.9	4.4	3.5	4.1	2.1	2.4	4.6	3.6
Chronic Pulmonary Disease	14.6	7.9	24.5	7.4	6.0	5.2	8.2	5.6	4.7
Pattern of Mortality									
Cumulative Mortality									
Days After Admission									
30	13.3%	25.5%	13.5%	7.6%	2.4%	3.1%	1.1%	4.7%	3.6%
90	22.5	30.7	20.2	12.6	4.7	5.9	3.0	6.5	7.8
180	29.9	34.4	25.2	17.3	6.7	8.2	5.5	8.1	12.7
270	35.5	37.2	29.0	20.8	8.6	9.6	7.5	9.2	15.5
360	41.0	39.4	32.7	24.3	10.0	11.3	9.7	9.3	17.8

Relative Risk of Dying[3]									
Female vs Male	0.77	(0.99)	0.71	0.82	0.69	0.62	--	(1.20)	0.72
Black vs Other Races	0.82	0.88	1.11	(0.93)	(1.26)	(1.29)	1.30	(1.57)	1.51
Age, 80 vs 65 years	1.50	1.85	1.89	1.81	2.77	3.90	3.14	1.79	1.43
Malignancy	2.25	1.46	2.97	5.17	6.30	3.80	3.26	2.36	2.21
Autoimmune Disease	(1.04)	(0.75)	(1.12)	(0.83)	(2.09)	(0.59)	(0.63)	(1.48)	(1.59)
Chronic Liver Disease	1.57	2.22	1.57	2.97	3.56	6.18	3.90	--	4.79
Chronic Renal Disease	2.14	2.16	2.58	2.95	9.68	5.88	2.65	4.74	2.46
Degenerative Cerebral Disease & Psychosis	(1.08)	0.72	1.28	1.46	2.48	2.14	2.35	--	(1.10)
Hypertensive Disease	0.67	0.63	0.61	0.59	(0.76)	0.65	0.64	0.59	0.53
Ischemic Heart Disease & Failure	--	--						--	--
Diabetes	(1.07)	1.15	1.22	1.37	1.38	1.98	1.49	(1.04)	(1.45)
Chronic Pulmonary Disease	(0.95)	(0.94)	0.89	1.19	1.67	1.79	1.62	(0.80)	(1.29)
Pattern of Morbidity									
Duration of Hospitalization[4]									
Primary Admission (days)	8.6/6.7	10.1/8.2	9.5/7.5	7.3/5.7	11.6/10.1	15.7/14.1	7.8/6.7	15.5/13.4	10.4/8.1
Primary and subsequent admissions (days)	16.2/11.0	15.2/11.1	14.8/10.3	12.4/8.2	14.0/11.4	19.6/16.6	10.9/8.3	19.2/15.8	15.0/10.6
Proportions of Patients with the Specified Number of Readmissions:[5]									
0	51.7%	55.5%	62.5%	65.3%	79.4%	75.2%	73.8%	68.1%	65.3%
1	26.0	26.5	22.9	21.6	14.1	18.8	18.4	21.7	21.4
2	11.9	10.4	8.1	7.4	4.3	4.3	4.7	6.9	8.2
3 or more	10.4	7.6	6.5	5.7	2.2	2.2	3.0	3.3	5.1
Causes of Readmissions[6]									
Pulmonary	11.1%	7.0%	34.5%	8.3%	8.3%	8.8%	8.5%	7.8%	7.3%
Cardiovascular	54.1	66.9	20.1	14.7	19.4	12.5	16.6	43.4	49.6
Gastrointestinal	8.1	6.9	10.2	38.7	27.2	11.2	11.9	10.7	10.0
Musculoskeletal	2.7	1.9	4.9	5.6	6.2	32.5	4.4	4.1	3.4
Genitourinary	4.6	3.2	5.7	5.6	6.7	5.3	28.3	5.0	4.4
Complications of treatment	0.8			0.8	0.8	2.6	4.4	0.9	0.4

Table 5.8 (continued)

	HFS	AMI	PNU	GIH	CSX	JTP	TUP	CAB	PCM
Patients with Prior[6] Admissions	33.2%	23.6%	29.3%	31.1%	29.4%	21.2%	22.0%	63.0%	33.6%
Causes of Prior Admissions									
Pulmonary	17.2%	8.8%	18.1%	19.6%	6.6%	6.8%	8.9%	2.2%	5.2%
Cardiovascular	32.7	43.7	19.4	10.1	17.4	12.2	18.8	86.3	56.5
Gastrointestinal	11.1	10.4	12.1	18.7	45.6	12.0	15.2	2.8	8.2
Musculoskeletal	5.3	5.7	8.4	9.2	5.3	32.6	5.0	1.2	3.5
Charges for Medical Care[4]									
Total, per patient	$10500/6500	$11600/7600	$9300/5900	$8500/5900	$10600/5300	$15900/13900	$8100/6300	$32200/28800	$18500/15900
Hospital Charges									
Primary Admission	4300	6100	4800	3800	7000	10200	4100	22700	12800
Primary and Readmissions	8600	9800	7700	6700	8500	12100	5900	25100	15500
Hospital-related Charges	900	1200	720	950	1700	2600	1600	6400	2100
Ambulatory Care[7]	640	460	570	570	350	540	520	630	620
Supportive Care[7]	280	150	310	240	100	710	90	140	160
Contributions to Charges (increment in dollars)[8]									
Female vs. Male	200	(-100)	-200	-200	(-30)	1500	-500	---	1200
Black vs. Other Races	300	-800	500	500	800	1900	1700	1100	3500
Age, 80 vs. 65	-1100	-1600	-200	-200	(-100)	1700	-500	1000	3300
Malignancy	(-400)	(0)	1400	1400	1400	4400	1900	2500	6500
Autoimmune Disease	(800)	(-400)	900	900	(-300)	(200)	(900)	1300	(1500)
Chronic Liver Disease	(-20)	(-1200)	(300)	(300)	3000	3100	5500	(600)	---
Chronic Renal Disease	2100	2000	2400	2400	4900	6100	11300	2600	14600
Degenerative Cerebral Disease & Psychosis	-700	(-600)	(100)	(100)	(10)	2600	-1500	2100	(3100)
Hypertensive Disease	-500	(-200)	-700	-700	-400	-900	-400	-300	-1100
Ischemic Heart Disease & Failure	---	---	700	700	800	1300	700	800	---
Diabetes	600	700	1000	1000	900	2300	(500)	1300	2300
Chronic Pulmonary Disease	600	900	1000	1000	1100	2200	600	1100	2800

Notes:

1., 2., and 3. As in Table 5.6.

4. Where two values separated by a "/" are given, the first is the arithmetic and the second the geometric mean.

5. The percentages are of patients at risk of readmission, i.e. of those discharged alive.

6. The causes were ascertained from the discharge diagnosis related group coded on the bill.

7. This consists of charges for Medicare-covered skilled nursing facility and home health agency services.

8. These quantities were computed from linear regression analyses of the logarithms of the charges accumulated in calendar year 1984 subsequent to the index admission. Additional covariates in the calculations resulting in the above data were: (1) number of beds in the hospital, (2) the ratio of interns to beds, (3) the 1984 HCFA wage index for the hospital, (4) whether the hospital was urban or rural. The base for the increments is the geometric mean of total charges. The increments in parentheses differed from 0 with a probability less than 90% (P > 0.1).

Table 5.9

Admissions during Calendar Year 1985: Outcomes of Care for Nine Selected Conditions or Procedures

	HFS	AMI	PNU	GIH	CSX	JTP	TUP	CAB	PCM
Percent of all patients hospitalized[1]	6.15%	4.53%	5.14%	2.29%	1.78%	2.43%	3.18%	1.03%	0.89%
Patient Characteristics									
Age: Under 65	6.4%	7.1%	7.4%	7.4%	8.6%	5.4%	3.5%	13.0%	3.5%
65-74	32.7	44.6	33.1	36.2	54.9	40.8	51.9	70.7	31.5
75-84	38.9	36.2	36.2	36.9	29.6	38.4	36.3	15.9	44.1
84 and over	22.0	12.1	23.4	19.4	6.9	15.4	8.3	0.5	20.9
Sex: Male	42.7%	46.7%	48.0%	44.4%	39.9%	29.4%	--	70.4%	47.2%
Race: White	86.6%	89.8%	89.5%	88.0%	91.3%	92.6%	89.6%	93.7%	91.0%
Black	9.9	6.2	7.0	8.4	4.4	4.0	6.6	2.4	6.1
Comorbidities[2]									
Malignancy	3.4%	1.5%	6.8%	5.2%	3.5%	1.7%	7.6%	0.8%	1.5%
Autoimmune Disease	1.0	0.7	1.4	1.8	0.7	2.1	0.2	0.4	0.4
Chronic Liver Disease	0.7	0.2	0.5	3.4	2.7	0.2	0.1	0	0.1
Chronic Renal Disease	5.3	2.5	2.3	3.1	0.7	0.6	1.1	1.1	1.7
Degenerative Cerebral Disease & Psychosis	1.7	1.2	3.7	2.4	0.9	2.1	0.8	0.3	1.5
Hypertensive Disease	14.5	17.5	9.7	12.8	16.0	18.5	11.3	19.1	18.2
Ischemic Heart Disease & Failure	--	--	36.6	25.7	21.9	19.5	18.3	--	--
Diabetes	9.4	8.6	5.2	4.4	5.0	2.5	2.8	5.6	4.8
Chronic Pulmonary Disease	17.3	9.2	27.2	8.6	7.1	6.0	8.7	6.4	6.1
Pattern of Mortality									
Cumulative Mortality									
Days After Admission									
30	13.7%	25.4%	14.3%	8.0%	2.6%	2.3%	1.0%	6.2%	3.2%
90	22.7	30.8	21.6	13.5	4.8	4.7	3.0	8.2	6.7
180	30.4	34.6	26.7	17.8	6.6	6.8	5.5	9.9	11.1
270	36.1	37.5	30.5	20.9	8.4	8.2	7.8	10.5	14.4
360	41.2	40.2	33.8	23.7	10.1	9.9	9.8	11.8	17.8

Relative Risk of Dying[3]

Female vs. Male	0.79	(0.96)	0.73	0.88	0.86	0.72	--	1.40	(0.89)
Black vs. Other Races	0.84	0.88	1.16	1.31	1.64	(1.12)	(1.16)	1.68	(0.89)
Age, 80 vs. 65 years	1.20	1.78	1.79	1.96	2.85	4.66	2.33	1.55	1.80
Malignancy	2.13	1.53	3.13	5.20	7.31	5.35	3.30	(1.23)	1.89
Autoimmune Disease	(1.16)	0.68	(0.97)	(0.91)	(0.79)	(1.37)	(2.34)	(0.82)	(1.65)
Chronic Liver Disease	(1.23)	(1.35)	2.34	3.39	3.04	4.19	--	--	--
Chronic Renal Disease	1.95	1.96	2.59	3.82	4.34	4.60	2.41	3.10	2.80
Degenerative Cerebral Disease & Psychosis	1.19	0.77	1.31	(1.16)	(1.51)	1.96	(1.66)	--	(1.27)
Hypertensive Disease	0.67	0.60	0.51	0.55	0.63	0.75	(0.80)	0.57	(0.94)
Ischemic Heart Disease & Failure	--	--	1.33	1.56	1.47	1.76	1.55	--	--
Diabetes	(1.01)	1.24	1.17	1.33	(1.14)	2.39	1.57	(1.00)	1.59
Chronic Pulmonary Disease	(1.01)	(0.95)	0.79	1.22	(1.24)	1.54	1.40	1.54	(1.15)

Pattern of Morbidity

Duration of Hospitalization[4]									
Primary Admission (days)	7.8/ 6.3	9.3/ 7.6	8.9/ 7.1	6.8/5.4	10.9/ 9.4	14.1/12.8	6.9/6.0	14.9/12.9	9.4/7.4
All Admissions (days)	14.8/10.1	14.0/10.4	13.7/ 9.7	11.4/7.8	13.4/10.7	17.6/15.0	9.7/7.4	17.8/14.7	13.6/9.7

Proportions of Patients with the Specified Number of Readmissions:[5]									
0	52.8%	55.8%	63.6%	66.7%	81.1%	75.8%	76.1%	72.0%	66.7%
1	26.5	27.0	22.1	20.7	13.1	18.0	16.1	19.6	20.6
2	11.3	10.2	8.4	7.2	3.6	4.2	4.8	5.5	7.8
3 or more	9.4	7.0	5.9	5.4	2.2	2.0	2.9	2.9	4.9

Causes of Readmissions[6]									
Pulmonary	11.3%	6.7%	34.1%	9.4%	10.0%	9.5%	9.8%	8.5%	8.5%
Cardiovascular	53.7	69.7	19.6	16.6	21.5	13.8	16.3	50.1	50.0
Gastrointestinal	7.9	6.0	10.1	37.0	27.7	8.6	12.0	11.2	9.0
Musculoskeletal	2.9	1.5	4.8	5.7	5.6	32.7	3.9	2.3	3.0
Genitourinary	5.0	2.9	6.1	5.5	7.2	5.9	27.2	4.9	5.0
Complications of treatment					0.8	1.5	4.7	0.8	1.0

Table 5.9 (continued)

	HFS	AMI	PNU	GIH	CSX	JTP	TUP	CAB	PCM
Patients with Prior[6] Admissions	32.6%	21.8%	28.0%	29.5%	26.7%	17.6%	21.3%	63.1%	32.5%
Causes of Prior Admissions									
Pulmonary	18.0%	10.5%	20.9%	11.6%	8.0%	8.4%	9.9%	2.0%	8.6%
Cardiovascular	35.5	44.5	21.0	20.0	19.6	14.6	20.6	86.5	59.4
Gastrointestinal	9.4	11.1	11.9	20.1	43.5	13.1	14.5	2.8	5.9
Musculoskeletal	5.5	5.1	7.6	8.4	4.0	32.9	5.9	1.3	4.2
Genitourinary	5.9	6.2	6.5	6.9	6.9	5.1	25.2	1.9	4.5
Charges for Medical Care[4]									
Total, per patient	$11000/7000	$12500/8100	$9800/6400	$8900/5700	$11500/8700	$16600/14500	$8300/6400	$34400/30200	$18900/16300
Hospital Charges									
Primary Admission	4400	6300	5000	3900	7500	10500	4100	24700	12800
Primary and Readmissions	8700	10300	7900	6900	9100	12400	5800	26800	15500
Hospital-related Charges	1000	1300	750	1000	1800	2700	1600	6700	2300
Ambulatory Care[7]	880	630	790	750	510	690	720	810	830
Supportive Care[7]	360	190	340	280	130	750	120	160	250
Contributions to Charges (increment in dollars)[8]									
Female vs Male	(100)	(-60)	-200	(-)	-1000	(-200)	--	2400	(500)
Black vs Other Races	400	-400	400	1400	2200	2200	1200	5100	3300
Age, 80 vs 65 years	-1100	-1700	-200	(-100)	2000	-500	1000·	3400	-600
Malignancy	(-100)	(-600)	1300	1400	4600	3100	2500	(3200)	2800
Autoimmune Disease	(60)	(-30)	1100	(600)	2900	2400	(400)	(300)	(-2800)
Chronic Liver Disease	1200	-1900	1200	2500	3700	4800	2700	--	(400)
Chronic Renal Disease	2600	2100	2400	3300	12700	4700	3533	18000	6700
Degenerative Cerebral Disease & Psychosis	-700	(-300)	(50)	(-400)	1900	-1300	1200	(600)	(-800)
Hypertensive Disease	-200	(40)	-700	-600	-1000	(-400)	-200	-3000	-1200
Ischemic Heart Disease & Failure	--	--	900	1100	1500	900	700	--	--
Diabetes	1300	600	1200	1600	1700	1700	1800	3600	1500
Chronic Pulmonary Disease	1100	1300	1300	1200	1900	1400	1000	2400	(400)

Notes:

1., 2., and 3. As in Table 5.6.

4. Where two values separated by a "/" are given, the first is the arithmetic and the second the geometric mean.

5. The percentages are of patients at risk of readmission, i.e of those discharged alive.

6. The causes were ascertained from the discharge diagnosis related group coded on the bill.

7. This consists of charges for Medicare-covered skilled nursing facility and home health agency services.

8. These quantities were computed from linear regression analyses of the logarithms of the charges accumulated in calendar year 1985 subsequent to the index admission. Additional covariates in the calculations resulting in the above data were: (1) number of beds in the hospital, (2) the ratio of interns to beds, (3) the 1984 HCFA wage index for the hospital, (4) whether the hospital was urban or rural. The base for the increments is the geometric mean of total charges. The increments in parentheses differed from 0 with a probability less than 90% ($P > 0.1$).

diagnoses such as benign prostatic hyperplasia (Stephen Jencks, private communication). On the other hand, diabetes, with similar effects, remains predictive of higher mortality.

Among the tracer conditions, a slight trend to higher mortality rates following hospitalization is apparent in the case of the medical admissions (see tables 5.8 and 5.9). No clear pattern is evident in the admissions for surgical procedures. The mortality rates following cholecystectomy, transurethral prostatectomy, and pacemaker implantation are very similar in the two years, whereas that following coronary artery bypass graft surgery is markedly higher, and that following major joint procedures, almost exclusively replacements of hips or knees, is markedly lower. In both instances, the actual number of procedures performed was higher in 1985 than in 1984, despite the general lowering of rates of admission. In the case of joint procedures, the lower mortality rate cannot be accounted for by an increased frequency of the lower-risk knee replacements (postoperative mortality rate, i.e., within 30 days of admission, of 0.6%) compared to hip replacements (postoperative mortality rate of 3.8%), the latter accounting for about two-thirds of the procedures in both years. The rise in the mortality rate in coronary artery bypass graft surgery may be related to an approximate doubling in the rate of percutaneous transluminal coronary angioplasty (data not shown).

As in the case of mortality, patients first admitted for medical conditions and for implantation of a permanent pacemaker tended to be readmitted more frequently and, thus, to consume more resources in charges and days of care than patients admitted for surgical procedures (see Table 5.7). In all time intervals, the organ system whose failure resulted in the index admission is also the most common cause of readmission. The highest probability of readmission occurs within the first 30 days of initial discharge, with 9–22% patients who survived the initial admission being readmitted. In the following 150 days, the rate drops to 3.7–9.3% per month, and levels off in the subsequent 180 days at 3.5–8.6% per month. Estimates based on the actuarial method indicate that, excluding readmissions on the day of discharge, within two years of discharge, 44–79% of the patients admitted with the tracer conditions will be readmitted at least once for all causes and 15–63% for causes related to the initial admission. The influence of comorbidities on the probability of readmission generally parallels that of mortality rates. The incidence of readmissions appears lower in 1985 than in 1984 for all the tracer conditions (see Tables 5.8 and 5.9). Because of incompleteness of the 1985 data, the reduction is overstated. However, as in the case of the aggregate populations, at least there is no indication of an increase in the incidence of readmissions.

Only a fifth to a third of the patients with an index admission in 1984 or 1985 had a prior admission except for those admitted for coronary bypass surgery. Of the latter, almost two-thirds had recent prior admissions of, usually, short duration in half of which cardiac catheterization was performed. If these presumably diagnostic admissions are excluded, the incidence of admissions for morbidity prior to bypass graft surgery falls to levels comparable to those in the other conditions.

Tables 5.8 and 5.9 also present the charges for the care of patients accumulated from the time of the first admission in the calendar year for the condition specified until the end of the year, i.e., over an average of six months. Although the charges for services provided by hospitals are virtually all covered, only about 60% of those billed by physicians and certain laboratories are allowed by the carriers of insurance acting as agents for the Health Care Financing Administration. These latter charges compose the component labeled ''Hospital-Related Charges'' and a portion of the charges for ''Ambulatory Care.'' In all, care delivered in hospital accounts for 88% or more of all Medicare-covered charges. Although they remain a small component of the total, the charges for supportive care of patients who had undergone replacement of hip or knee joints stand out. They are comparable in magnitude to those incurred by patients hospitalized for stroke (data not shown). The increment in overall charges from 1984 to 1985 is quite small, 2–8%, but must be viewed in the context of the reductions of comparable proportion in the durations of both the initial and all the hospitalizations during the period of follow-up. The increment in charges for ambulatory care is proportionately large (30–40%) but small in absolute terms ($150–210) per hospitalized patient. This increase is slightly overstated because data on about 4% of the bills that determine all the hospital-related and about half the ambulatory-care charges for 1984 were lost.

The influence of demographic characteristics and comorbidities on costs is highly variable. The presence of chronic renal, pulmonary, liver, and cardiac disease and of diabetes generally results in higher charges. The influence of hypertensive disease as a comorbidity, after allowance is made for the presence of the other comorbidities, is similar in the case of charges to its influence on mortality, i.e., negative. Caution must be exercised in the interpretation of the increments of cost or risk of death due to the less-frequent comorbidities such as malignancy in coronary artery bypass graft surgery because the estimates of the increments are based on relatively few cases.

DISCUSSION

The objective of the present analyses was to establish a baseline against which to monitor the evolution of medical practices in the United States and to begin to assess the impact of the major administrative changes in the Medicare program that occurred at the end of 1983 and during 1984. It is important to assess the impact of the conversion to a prospective modified fixed-price payment system and the establishment of the peer review organizations to assure the appropriateness and effectiveness of the care provided in hospitals.

External verification of the accuracy of data currently available to HCFA cannot be readily accomplished principally because of substantial differences in

case-selection methodology between the present and previously published reports. The population studied herein is an essentially random sample of all
hospitalized Medicare beneficiaries rather than patients of specific centers. In
addition, the specific tracer conditions were selected on the basis of diagnosis-
related group classifications assigned as a result of ICD–9–CM diagnosis and
procedure codes entered by the hospitals on the bills submitted to HCFA, a
procedure made possible by the introduction of DRGs to determine reimbursements in fiscal 1984. Thus, uniformly lower estimates of postsurgery mortality
rates were obtained in the present analyses than in the work of Riley and Lubitz
(1985) on procedures performed in 1979–1980 on Medicare patients over 65 on
a database most nearly comparable to the present one. In most instances the
differences are small and may be partly due to improvements in technique and
partly to the inclusion of Medicare patients under 65 as well as the use of the
actuarial method to compute cumulative mortality rates in the present but not in
the previous work. That changes in coding practices are occurring is also suggested by the higher frequency of comorbidities in patients admitted in 1985
than in 1984, although some of this may also be due to selection only of more
severely ill patients for admissions in 1985.

However, if the data available to the federal government are accepted as valid,
they indicate that criteria for admission are highly responsive to administrative
constraints. The principal objective of the peer review organizations in their first
contract period (late 1984–late 1986) was the control of hospital admission rates.
In view of the change in case mix and, most dramatically, in postadmission
mortality rates from 1984 to 1985 that suggest, in addition, a shift to higher
severity of illness within diagnostic categories, this objective has been achieved.
Whether this is ascribable to the activities of the PROs and/or the Prospective
Payment System or simply reflects a continuing trend in medical practice cannot
be certain. However, the stability of postadmission mortality rates in 1983–1984
and the substantial increase in 1985 does imply an impact of the more recent
interventions. On the other hand, analysis of the tracer conditions does indicate
that the effectiveness of the medical care provided to Medicare beneficiaries has
not been compromised: no substantial deterioration in outcomes, i.e., in mortality, morbidity, disability rates, or costs is evident. The two conditions in
which large differences in postadmission mortality rates are observed tend to
support this conclusion. In both instances the absolute number of first admissions
was higher in 1985 than in 1984, while, in general, admission rates decreased
substantially. In the case of major joint procedures, the postoperative mortality
rate decreased, while in the case of coronary artery bypass graft surgery, it
increased. In the absence of more detailed information about the characteristics
of the patients and the nature of the care provided, the causes for these changes
can only be speculated upon. However, the government and the peer review
organizations are undertaking projects at present to obtain more complete data
on selected samples of patients admitted for conditions of interest to permit a

more exhaustive analysis of the factors that influence outcomes, as has already been done in the case of renal transplantation (Krakauer, 1986).

Relative to the focus of this volume, it seems reasonable to conclude from the data reviewed here that, at least in this initial period under study, Medicare-based changes in hospital patient-care practices and use of technology did not have a negative impact on patient outcomes. Continuing assessments will be needed to determine whether this situation prevails in the future.

ACKNOWLEDGMENTS

The assistance and advice of the staff of the Division of Data Development, Bureau of Data Management and Strategy, HCFA, in particular I. Goldstein, J. Welsh, D. I. Swaner, M. P. Clifford, and M. Sheppard, are very much appreciated and gratefully acknowledged. Dr. B. A. McCann and P. Brooks were most helpful in the identification and coding of the comorbidities. Special thanks are due Dr. D. W. Alling of the National Institute of Allergy and Infectious Diseases for a careful and critical reading of the manuscript.

APPENDIX

High Risk	Diagnosis	ICD-9-CM Codes*
CA	Cancer	141-160, 162-172, 174-209
CE	Stroke	430-432, 434, 436
HS	Severe acute heart disease	410, 427.1,. 427.4, 427.5, 441.0, 441.1, 441.3, 441.5, 441.9,785.51
HM	Severe chronic heart disease	398.91, 402.01, 402.11, 402.91, 425, 428, 518.4
GC	Gastrointestinal catastrophes	551, 557, 560.0, 560.2-560.9, 570, 572-572.7, 573.4, 567, 578.0, 578.9
ME	Metabolic and electrolyte	250.01-250.4, 251.0, 251.1,disorders255.4,, 276
PN	Pulmonary disease	415.1, 416.0, 480-483, 485- 516, 518-519, except 516.1, and 518.4
RN	Renal disease	580-590 except 580.81, and 590.81
SE	Sepsis	DRG:416, 417
TR	Severe	806, 808.43, 808.53, 820., 821, 828, 850.2, 850.4.., 851.1-851.7, 852, 839.0-839.5, 860-867, 887, 897, 900.0, 901-904, 926, 927.0, 928.0, 929.0, 942.3, 942.4, 942.5, 946.3-946.9, 947.1-947.9, 948.2-948.9, 952, 958.0, 958.1 958.4, 958.5

Low Risk		
EY	Ophthalmologic disease	360-379
GY	Gynecologic disease	617-629
HL	Low risk heart disease	393-429, except 415.1 and416.0 and cases in categories HS and HM

68

GI	Gastrointestinal disease	530-579, except 577.0, 573.1, and 573.2 and cases in category GC
GU	Urologic disease	593-609
OP	Orthopedic conditions	712-739, 810-838, 840-848 (excluding cases in category TR)
UN	All other Conditions	All other ICD-9-CM codes

All of the above entries refer to ICD-9-CM codes except for the entries for Sepsis which are expressed in terms of diagnosis=related groups (DRGs).

COMORBIDITY	ICD-9-CM CODES
Cancer	141-160.9, 162-172.9, 174-208.9
Chronic liver diseas	571-572.8
Chronic renal disease	582-583.9, 585-587
Chronic cardiovascular disease	412-414.9, 426-429.1
Chronic pulmonary disease	491-493.9, 496
Cerebrovascular degeneration/ chronic psychosis	290-290.9, 294-299.9
Hypertensive disease	402-405.99, 412-414.9
Diabetes	250.01, 250.1-250.9

(A comorbidity is taken to be present if its ICD-9-CM code appears on the bill as any one of the up to four additional diagnoses beyond the principal diagnosis.)

PART II
TECHNOLOGY AND THE HEALTH CARE ORGANIZATION

6

The Adoption and Diffusion of Process Technology by Industrial Organizations: Insights for the Health Care Industry?

Stephen R. Rosenthal

This chapter summarizes salient points about the adoption and diffusion of process technology in industrial settings in order to stimulate discussion of this topic by those in the health care field. The material presented here is drawn from the author's extensive research in the field of factory automation as well as from recent literature.

A major premise of this chapter is that health care managers, facing competition in their own industry, will increasingly look to new process technology as a potential competitive weapon and that they would benefit from insights drawn from their industrial counterparts. We must recognize from the start, however, that the health care industry differs in several critical structural respects from manufacturing industries. Accordingly, what is presented here is simply a starting point for the development of a comparable understanding of the potential processes for enhancing the adoption and diffusion of new technology in hospitals and other health care delivery settings. Completing such an analysis for the health care industry is beyond the scope of this chapter. In fact, given the new modes of competition in this industry and the many ways in which process technology can affect the cost and performance of health care delivery, it is an excellent topic for applied research and normative insights.

The perspective of this chapter is that of operations management. Accordingly, an emphasis is placed on the set of decisions regarding the acquisition and use of new process technology. This perspective is offered in the belief that in health care as well as other industries, successful innovation in process technology requires that someone (or some group) take the operations management perspective and, furthermore, that this perspective is best accomplished by thinking of technological innovation within the strategic context of a firm and the industry within which it must compete.

DECISIONS ABOUT NEW INDUSTRIAL TECHNOLOGY

We must distinguish between product technology and process technology. Pieces of equipment, such as a computer, a robot, or a machine tool, are products that need to be designed, developed, and produced. Such products can be examined to reveal their individual components and the connections among those components. One can readily ask and answer the questions: What technologies are embodied in this product? How do these technological capabilities translate into the performance characteristics of the product? How do they affect its cost? What were the critical trade-off decisions between higher performance and lower cost in the design of this product?

Now consider what happens when a collection of these same products—computers, robots, and machine tools—are brought together in a factory that makes, for example, jet engines. To the jet-engine producer, these pieces of equipment are process technologies (rather than product technologies) since they constitute part of the productive process through which components of the jet engine are fabricated.

The notions of product technology and process technology are not confined to the world of manufacturing. In a service industry, such as health care, products (which embody particular technologies) become part of the process through which a patient is diagnosed or treated. A CT scanner is a central piece of process technology for a wide range of diagnostic activities. A renal dialysis unit is an example of process technology for caring for those with kidney failure.

The basic distinction, then, between product and process technology derives from one's point of view. The supplier of a piece of equipment sees it as a product to be designed, developed, and sold. The user of the technology sees it as the process, or means, through which another product gets developed or service gets delivered. Health care practitioners and managers typically deal with decisions about new process technology. The scope of those decisions is outlined below, and a summary of current practice is presented in the following section.

Types of Decisions on Process Innovation

Six types of decisions affect a company's innovation through new process technology. The first is *strategic planning* where senior management, aided perhaps by corporate staff, formulate a vision of how and why the company must be strong in its production processes if it is to succeed in the marketplace. The second is *operations planning* where manufacturing management and senior technical people try to define feasible bounds on the rate and direction of change in process technology. The third is *technology assessment* when engineering and operations managers review key technologies looking for those types that have the greatest change of providing the needed production capabilities. Next comes *technology selection* when teams of technical staff and procurement specialists decide on the particular version of the needed technology. After that are a series of decisions involving the *implementation* of the new technology. Here, operations managers, joined perhaps by supervisors and production workers, make choices that affect the company's initial installation of that process technology. The final set of decisions are made when corporate staff along with existing and potential users of the technology deal with issues of *technology transfer*.

Strategic Planning

Successful companies take strategic planning seriously. Even though the huge corporate staff groups engaged in this function in the 1970s have been all but eliminated throughout U.S. industry, strong senior management must think about issues such as the following:

- What is the company (or business unit) trying to accomplish? Given the market being pursued, what are the most important attributes of its products or services?
- Can the company achieve its objectives with existing process technologies? This is a complex question forcing management to project trends in competitive activity as well as to establish the performance limitations of its own current process technology.
- Is new technology available that might offer competitive advantages? Technical experts may have to join with those sensitive to emerging market demand and customer expectations in seeking an answer to this question.
- What should be the basis for justifying new technology of this type? Senior management should specify appropriate time horizons and evaluation criteria. Recently, the limits of traditional return on investment criteria for answering strategic questions of technology acquisition have been acknowledged, but this area still calls for explicit managerial articulation.

If strategic planning decisions are made with care, the stage is set for the next step, operations planning. If not, then the context for doing operations planning will be lacking.

Operations Planning

Operations planning as it relates to manufacturing is often an ongoing activity. Here we will concentrate on the technology-related aspects of this activity in which manufacturing managers periodically review the capabilities of their facilities to project how future production requirements will be met. Capital budgets provide the vehicle for planning the allocation of funds for needed process technology. Initial ideas for the technology to be acquired emerge from the efforts of groups of technical and managerial employees who attempt to answer questions such as the following:

- What kinds of changes do we need to make in the way our current products are manufactured?
- What kinds of new processing capabilities are going to be required when we begin to manufacture new products that are currently in the early planning stages?
- How fast must we proceed in enhancing our current production capabilities?
- How much senior management attention must be given to planning and executing such changes in process technology?
- How much support (human resources and capital) can we expect our organization to provide?

When questions such as these have been resolved, the company is ready to move beyond the operations planning stage to the more specific step of selecting particular new technologies to adopt. To do this successfully, the company needs to have been active in the assessment of technology.

Technology Assessment

Technology assessment in manufacturing is usually done by experts with titles such as manufacturing engineer or process engineer and is most common in companies that realize that new process technology is likely to offer them a competitive edge in the future. The types of generic questions that they would explore are:

- What functional value (e.g., precision, flexibility, capacity, reliability) is embodied in newly emerging process technology?
- How much risk (technological, economic) is currently inherent in these latest process technologies?
- How are these aspects of risk likely to decline in the next few years as more manufacturers gain experience in their use and as suppliers refine existing versions of the technology?
- How long will it be before such current "leading-edge" technology becomes seriously obsolete in the face of yet another "generation" of new technology?

These are admittedly very difficult questions to answer. The job of those assigned to the technology assessment function, however, is to develop the best insights they can, given the resources they have and the state of technological development in their field. Rough and partial answers are more helpful to those who need to select new process technology than none at all.

Technology Selection and Procurement

Large manufacturing organizations have the classic "make or buy" decision with respect to new process technology. Those with extensive process engineering or computer staff may have adequate capabilities to design and even develop some of the new technology needed to produce their own products. In fact, throughout the industrial history of the United States, many new technological developments came from companies that started out to improve their own operations (Rosenberg, 1976).[1] In the health care industry there is usually not much of an issue regarding "make or buy": health care providers tend to look to their traditional suppliers for new process technology, so purchased technology is by far the predominant situation.

In this mode of acquisition, vendor selection is very important, particularly in terms of the following decisions:

- How detailed must we be in providing operational specifications to our suppliers of new process technology?
- Who in our organization should participate in the selection of a supplier and, more significantly, in the selection of the technology to be purchased?
- What are the most important criteria (and priority order) to guide us in the selection among competing suppliers and technologies?
- What role should our "users" (hands-on production personnel) play in this procurement process?

Implementation

Selection is the first step in the adoption of new process technology since it includes decisions on what is needed, what it will cost, and who will supply it. Next comes the critical step of implementation—bringing it in and making it work. At this important juncture a new set of issues arises:

- Who should be in charge of the implementation process?
- How fast should we go from initial exposure and testing of the new process technology to its use in actual production mode?
- How much effort (and resources) must we allow for the start-up of the new technology?
- Will there be new or modified job requirements, and how will we design and implement them?
- What training requirements are inherent in the successful use of the new technology, and who will provide such training?

Such questions are likely to require careful consideration and may lead to considerable controversy, particularly if the new technology is radically different from the current approach to production operations. It is not at all unusual for a carefully conceived strategy for new process technology coupled with an elaborate effort in technology selection to falter due to an inadequate implementation plan or the casual execution of such a plan.

Technology Transfer

Having successfully implemented a new process technology in one of its plants, a manufacturer may well wish to do something similar in another plant. In health care, this is analogous to the multihospital organization or even the hospital with more than one category of service that might benefit from having the same new process technology. In the literature of technological innovation, this is called the stage of *technology transfer*, and it is characterized by the following kinds of questions:

• How much transfer should we attempt?
• What is the best sequence of transfer sites?
• How fast should we move to transfer this technology?
• How will we seek to accomplish the transfer process?

As with the other stages of technological innovation, knowing the questions to ask is only the beginning of the task in the transfer of technology. In many ways it is like starting all over again with implementation.

OBSERVATIONS ON RECENT EXPERIENCE WITH INDUSTRIAL PROCESS INNOVATION

The preceding section of this chapter presented a conceptual map of the various stages of industrial process innovation along with a list of the kinds of questions and issues that would be pursued at each of these stages. The purpose of this section is to summarize briefly what typically occurs at each of the stages. This is a look at practice as distinguished from theory (Rosenthal, 1984; Graham & Rosenthal, 1986; Leonard-Barton & Deschamps, 1989; Twiss, 1974).[2]

Strategic Planning

Answers to the strategic planning questions will only rarely be found in written form. Even when strategic planning is a formal activity, process technology is rarely included in any meaningful detail. Furthermore, process technology is generally poorly understood by senior management, very few of whom have spent any appreciable part of their careers within the manufacturing function.

Technological forecasting is a primitive art. Those who spend the most time trying to do it tend to be technologists themselves, and they often have an implicit optimism as to the rate of progress of new technologies that are just on the horizon.

There is much after-the-fact justification of radically new process technology. It is difficult to quantify all of the benefits, especially those that are more strategic in nature. This leads to a short-term bias in the justifications that are performed.

Unfortunately, many U.S. manufacturers cannot afford to wait until the justification numbers look better for new process technology. The pressing competitive need for improved quality and shortened production lead times force manufacturers, even in sophisticated companies, to take a "leap of faith" in adopting new process technology even before they can formally apply their own justification criteria.

Operations Planning

Manufacturers who have outstanding reputations spend considerable time on operations planning. However, much of this effort is in the area of capacity planning, while only a minority routinely tries to answer the questions about new processing capabilities. Senior management typically leaves to process engineers the planning of technological change. Typically, companies underestimate both the human resources, capital, and elapsed time necessary to accomplish a significant change in process technology.

Technology Assessment

Technology assessment is usually an afterthought. Under the pressure of solving today's production problems, not many manufacturers routinely spend enough time and effort monitoring emerging process technology. While they might know something about a new technology, it is not likely to be at the required level of specificity: functional value, full cost implications, and inherent risk.

Knowing the likely life cycle of existing leading-edge process technology is difficult to forecast. Suppliers of this technology often develop the next generation of the technology, thereby rendering their own products obsolete. However, these suppliers might wait to see how the current technology is doing in the marketplace before determining their own rate of product innovation.

Technology Selection and Procurement

Manufacturers often do not play a key role in the specification of the process technology that they wish to acquire from an outside supplier. Instead, they often look to the supplier to solve certain (poorly specified) operational requirements in the design of new technology. Sophisticated manufacturers have learned that it is a mistake to procure a complex system of new process technology on a "turnkey" basis, in which the manufacturer simply pays the bill when the system is installed and does not have to worry about either its detailed specification or its development. Instead, users must play a very active role in procurement if they are to get process technology that is appropriate for their production requirements.

Participation on procurement teams varies with company style. A small team of crossfunctional experts is likely to be more effective than a large team of specialists who have trouble understanding each others' points of view and technical concerns. Project management of procurement teams is very critical, and many companies lack people with significant skills in leading such teams.

Implementation

In implementing new process technology, technical experts often want to retain control over testing it. They thus resist pressure to hand it over to those who have ongoing production responsibilities. For this reason and others (including unanticipated operational complexities), startups last much longer than usually anticipated. Especially disturbing are the surprises that come from changes in job design and in the identification of new training requirements. The type of training that is offered by technology suppliers is usually designed to handle predictable technical situations as distinguished from the more subtle contextual difficulties of using the new technology in a particular production setting. In short, the implementation of new complex process technology in industrial settings is anything but routine.

Technology Transfer

Technology transfer is the diffusion of technology throughout an organization that has already adopted it for an initial application. Decentralized organizations often treat diffusion as an afterthought. Even sophisticated companies tend to underestimate the complexity of the technology transfer process. Technology transfer is very similar to initial implementation in that the follow-up adoption sites need to understand the need for the technology and to conduct the requisite planning and execution tasks. Selling key actors at the follow-up sites on the value of the new technology is a critical though often-neglected part of technology diffusion.[3] Perhaps the biggest single obstacle to successful technology diffusion is the mistaken assumption on the part of senior management that it should be much easier than the initial implementation project.

CONCLUSIONS

Innovation in process technology involves hierarchical sets of decisions in industrial organizations. These decisions are partly in the realm of senior management, but many others are routinely delegated to technical staff and different levels of operating personnel. It is unlikely that such decisions are well articulated in advance. Nor is it safe to assume that decisions on related issues are internally consistent or even well understood by all who are likely to be affected. In short, the management of technological innovation, from strategic planning through procurement, implementation, and technology transfer is not a well-developed function in most manufacturing organizations in the United States.

Industrial process technologies are complex in two senses. First, the technologies, typically computer-based, contain inherent *systems complexities*. Combinations of electronic and mechanical components, software plus hardware capabilities, makes it difficult for a manufacturer to feel comfortable that he or she knows what the technology is and what it is capable of producing. Second, the technology is itself embodied in a productive organization that generates *contextual complexity*. Knowing how to use the technology, how to respond to unforeseen problems, and how to manage the combined sociotechnical system for maximum performance presents a new set of managerial challenges.

Information on new leading-edge process technology is often inadequate. Suppliers are key actors, but they do not have all of the desired answers. Users and suppliers often must learn by doing in an informal partnership while attempting the initial adoption of such new process technology. Once this is accomplished, users still face significant managerial challenges in promoting the successful transfer of the new technology to other applications throughout the company.

What all this might mean for the health care industry, facing its own competitive pressures and technological opportunities, is the subject of another future paper. In reflecting on how the stages of innovation and experience from manufacturing might apply to the world of health care, one ought to consider the following points:

- Strategic planning and operational planning can be done in health care organizations, but they are likely to have a similar set of problems to those of organizations in other industries.

- Technology assessment for health care is not radically different from other fields.

- Technology selection and procurement will differ in three major respects: (1) the payers (insurers) and regulators make the process of selection more complex, (2) health care professionals (doctors) rather than senior managers are key decision makers, and (3) the medical equipment industry may be more likely independently to try to push new technology on its user industry than are the suppliers of manufacturing technology (who often wait for their customers to demonstrate a need for some new technological capability).

- Initial implementation success and subsequent technology transfer depend critically on doctor acceptance but are also subject to many of the general issues observed in the manufacturing setting.

The adoption and diffusion of process technology by industrial organizations certainly offers insights for those concerned with similar phenomena in the health care industry. Nevertheless, health care in the United States has certain distinguishing characteristics. Health care administrators would do well to appreciate the lessons learned from their industrial counterparts and then redefine the challenges and opportunities in terms of their own industry. Doing this may turn out to be difficult. Not to try is to invite disaster.

NOTES

1. Rosenberg (1976) presents historical examples of this phenomenon with respect to the machine tool industry. More recently, we find companies like McDonnel-Douglas and Lockheed in the aerospace industry and Tandy in the computer equipment industry, having pioneered in the development of computer-aided tools to aid their own design and manufacturing organizations, have turned these products into commercial ventures by selling them as process innovations for other manufacturing companies in many different industries.

2. This section does not pretend to be a complete summary of the literature. It is based largely on the author's own consulting experience and research on the management of factory automation technology (see, for example, Rosenthal, 1984; Graham & Rosenthal, 1986), other recent work (such as that of Leonard-Barton & Deschamps, 1989), and such literature as that of Twiss, 1974 (on technology transfer). Since this chapter is written for practitioners rather than researchers, I have not attempted to tie each observation to particular citations in the literature.

3. Leonard-Barton and Deschamps have studied this phenomenon and provide more detailed insights on the technology transfer phenomenon within large organizations.

7

Decision-Making for Technology:
The Hospital Perspective

Peter W. Van Etten

This chapter presents a hospital administrator's view of the prospects for the application of new technology in the radically altering health care environment. Before making predictions of my own, let me recall some of the predictions of the past few years that have not come true:

1. *The Prospective Payment System (PPS) would result in increased admissions.* Whereas admissions for the elderly had risen inexorably since Medicare began in 1966, starting in 1983, when PPS was implemented, admissions began declining despite the obvious incentive for hospitals to increase admissions. Medicare admissions were growing on an average of 4% a year, and over a five-year period (1979–1983), admissions increased 20%. In 1983, Medicare admissions reached a high of 11.8 million. After the implementation of PPS, Medicare admissions began to decline, starting in 1984 with 11.7 million admissions and dropping to 10.1 million in 1987. The number of Medicare enrollees has been increasing by 2% every year, and in 1987 there were 32.4 million elderly on the Medicare program.

2. *HMOs would be the dominant insurer by 1990.* HMOs have indeed made significant progress, but nowhere near the progress that many observers predicted 10 years ago. Even when all managed-care insurers are taken into account, it would seem that fee-for-service medicine is definitely here to stay for a significant portion of the population. National data suggest that 11.8% of the total population was enrolled in HMOs in 1987. In Massachusetts, the enrollment in managed-care plans is noticeably higher, with 20.4%. The number

of elderly enrolled in HMOs on a national basis has also grown. In 1986 approximately 4.5% of the Medicare population was enrolled in HMOs while only three years earlier the enrollment was 1.9% of the Medicare population. The Massachusetts percentages mirror the national statistics for Medicare enrollees in managed-care plans.

3. *Teaching hospitals will be big losers in a competitive environment.* In many metropolitan areas, such as Boston, New York, Philadelphia, and Chicago, teaching-hospital admissions have either increased or decreased far less than each area's community hospitals despite the fact that teaching-hospital costs for treating similar patients are often double that of community hospitals. A brief analysis using American Hospital Association data shows that community hospitals vary more in admissions and occupancy than teaching hospitals. In California, most teaching hospitals are very profitable.

4. *Price will be the primary concern of payers and hospital managers.* Instead, payers are increasingly concerned about quality and availability of services. These concerns are due primarily to market pressures upon payers from subscribers.

5. *Declines in occupancy will result in widespread closure of hospitals.* Instead, many hospitals, including most of the large chains, have managed to maintain or increase their profitability despite occupancy rates at or below 50%. Obviously hospital costs are a good deal more variable than many people once predicted.

6. *DRGs and competition will radically alter decision-making for technology in hospitals.* Since this is the major issue for consideration here, I will not offer an immediate rebuttal but rather first review some of the changes currently taking place within the health care environment, and then offer some examples from hospitals as to how decision-making is changing regarding the application of new technology in health care.

The Prospective Payment System has had an enormous impact upon hospitals. The primary impact of PPS, however, is due less to the introduction of DRGs than to significantly altered rates of payment. The rates have changed every year since the inception of PPS. Aside from various blending problems between hospital-specific rates and national rates, the Health Care Financing Administration (HCFA) has not allowed sufficient increases for inflation. The rates usually provide for minimal or no inflation. In addition, the DRGs are recalibrated every year, and new weights are assigned, thus changing the reimbursement for a given procedure. Another issue specific to teaching hospitals is the decline in the indirect medical education component of the rate over the last few years. It is thus the shift in the level of overall payments rather than the method of payment that has resulted in changed hospital behavior, together with the increasingly effective activities of PROs. Many of the predictions regarding the changes in medical practice that would result from DRGs have not taken place. Certainly there is greater attention to length of stay. But beyond this one crude aspect of per-case cost I doubt that there have been widespread changes in medical practice.

At this point most hospitals still lack even rudimentary reporting information regarding the marginal profitability of their Medicare patients. Even if they did have this information, most hospital administrators are unwilling to try to coerce or coax physicians into changing medical practice. Instead, many administrators are desperately trying to fill empty beds. This is not to say that technical issues affecting DRG computation, such as the amount of the discrete adjustment factor or the lag time in recalibration, are not important issues that need more scrutiny. However, I do not feel that these issues will have specific impact upon hospital decision-making.

An issue more important than DRGs that directly affects medical decision-making is the treatment of capital expenses under the Prospective Payment System. Despite two years of strenuous efforts by the Reagan administration, capital still remains a pass through. As a result, the one remaining cost-plus aspect of hospital reimbursement is the payment of capital expenses, including, of course, those for technology. Congress has indeed made arbitrary reductions of first 7% and then 10% from capital payments. However, hospitals still have significant incentives to substitute capital for labor and to adopt new technology with little regard for cost-benefit issues, at least as far as Medicare reimbursement is concerned. When capital is indeed included within the DRG payment or capped, there may be significant changes in the application of technology.

While DRGs may not yet have had a significant impact upon hospital decision-making, the introduction of market forces has indeed had a significant impact. Managed-care plans that solicit bids from hospitals based upon price still represent a minority of patients in most of the nation's hospitals. However, even when only 5% of the hospital's patients are derived from HMOs or PPOs, there is often a significant impact on the hospital's behavior. Few hospitals explicitly treat one group of patients differently from another. Therefore the concern for costs for only 5% of a hospital's patients often has a far greater impact upon all of the hospital's patients. Often, however, the financial incentives inherent in treating managed-care patients run counter to financial incentives for Medicare patients. Most contracts for managed-care patients are on a per-diem basis introducing a set of incentives quite contrary to that of case-based payment. In California, hospitals are paid by different payers on the basis of charges, per diems, and DRGs. The financial incentives of one form of payment are canceled out by another.

Probably a more important issue for hospital administrators than whether they are paid by DRGs or by HMOs is that there is an increasing scarcity of patients. American Hospital Association data indicate that inpatient admissions started to decline on a national basis for short-term nonfederal hospitals as early as 1981. The number of admissions went from 36.5 million in 1981 to 32.4 million in 1986. Conversely, outpatient visits have increased as expected from 206 million in 1981 to 234 million in 1986. The average length of stay has held steady for almost seven years at 7.6 days. In 1984 the average dropped to 7.3 days, and in 1985 and 1986 the average dropped to 7.1 days. Occupancy has also declined;

in 1981 it was 75.9% nationally, and by 1986 it had gone down to 64.2%. The utilization statistics for Massachusetts show the same trend at a slightly slower rate. As length of stay and admissions decline, the most critical issue faced by hospital administrators is to somehow fill beds. Once the bed is full, the administrator can worry about how much payment will be received. Only third on the list of critical concerns is the issue of the cost of treating the patient. Occupancy is a much more critical factor in survival for most institutions than payment rates or cost effectiveness. As a result, the primary factor determining most hospital administrators' decision-making regards issues of strategic planning and marketing to increase activity.

Anne Greer studied decision-making regarding medical technology in 25 hospitals between 1976 and 1980 (Greer, forthcoming). She determined that there were three categories of decisions made within health care institutions:

1. *Decisions regarding the availability and use of immediate clinical tools used in diagnosis and treatment.* She found that these decisions were usually made by physicians either individually or in peer groups and were rarely questioned by administrators.

2. *Decisions regarding the introduction and use of service department technologies such as radiology and laboratory.* She found that financial issues were of some concern, and decisions for this category involved the participation of both administration and clinicians.

3. *Decisions regarding the range and availability of services such as heart programs or obstetrics.* She found predominant involvement by administrators and governing boards for this third type of decision-making.

In the nine years since the end of Greer's study, significant changes have occurred in hospital decision-making regarding investment in medical technology. The typology of the past has become blurred. Decision-making in most hospitals involves the integration of a number of criteria including financial issues, quality concerns, impact upon public awareness of the institution, as well as the traditional need to satisfy physician interests. This integration now takes place for all the categories of decisions that Greer identified. Integration implies decision-making at a higher level of the organization than was the case previously. However, this is not to suggest that chief executive officers of hospitals make all decisions regarding medical technology. Instead, decision-making at the top is increasingly shared with physicians. Indeed, administrative structures of hospitals represent a broader spectrum of disciplines and interests than was true in the past.

Here are 10 examples of decisions made regarding the investment in technology at teaching hospitals around the country, illustrating the complex interrelationship of issues in regard to the implementation of new technology:

1. *Implantable Defibrillators.* This program is a financial loser since most third parties will not pay for this procedure. A decision was made to implement the program, although on a limited basis, primarily because it was felt that this program could strengthen the referrals for the hospital's cardiology service, which

is quite a profitable service. Therefore, it was deemed prudent to approve a program that itself lost money because of the expectation that other programs' profitable activity would increase.

2. *Bone Marrow Transplants.* This program also is a financial loser. The decision was made to embark slowly upon the program since it would strengthen the hospital's oncology program. Unlike cardiology, oncology is not a profitable service at present. This is largely a result of the inadequacy of DRGs in identifying the higher severity of oncology patients treated at teaching hospitals than in community hospitals. While oncology is not presently profitable, the hospital determined that in the long run oncology was a very important service that might become profitable, particularly as the hospital developed new means of contracting with payers to pay for an entire episode of illness rather than a single oncology encounter. So the decision with regard to bone marrow transplant was based upon a belief that financial and programmatic benefits to the hospital would eventually result despite immediate short-run losses.

3. *Interleukin 2.* Most of this new program's expense was covered by research grants; however, there was a significant portion that would have to be billed to the patient and would probably involve bad debts. The program was undertaken because of the hospital's commitment to clinical research and, also, because it was felt that the prestige that would result from the program would increase referrals for many services.

4. *Liver Transplantation.* In one case, extensive efforts were made in negotiations with the state and other payers to ensure that payment for liver transplantation would equal marginal costs. In the end these efforts were not successful, yet the program was still established. Primary reasons for undertaking the program were that the hospital had made a strong commitment to expand transplantation in the belief that organ transplantation would be an important part of tertiary hospital-care activity in the years to come. In particular, it was felt that whereas many tertiary services that had been introduced in the teaching hospital were soon duplicated in community hospitals, transplantation would remain a service offered only by a few specialized institutions and could therefore enable the hospital to establish a distinct identity in the marketplace. The introduction to the program was done on a collaborative basis with three other teaching hospitals, largely because of the influence of the certificate of need program.

5. *Angioplasties.* While the reimbursement for angioplasties is quite favorable, profitability is less than for bypass, the alternative surgical treatment. The hospital embarked upon the program because the hospital's cardiologists believe that the angioplasty program would enable them to gain increased referrals; also, the hospital's competitors had already established angioplasty programs, and the cardiologists believed that a less-invasive procedure was of benefit to patients.

6. *New Intensive Care Unit Beds.* Reimbursement for intensive care unit (ICU) beds is now undifferentiated from other payment, so the addition of 11 very expensive new beds would, in most cases, result in a financial loss. In this case, however, since a certificate of need was obtained, all of the capital and

operating costs associated with ICU beds were passed on to third-party payers, with, of course, the exception of fixed-price contracts with HMOs. The intensive care unit beds emphasize the hospital's strategic decision to emphasize its tertiary services rather than secondary services.

7. *Magnetic Resonance Imaging (MRI)*. Despite the fact that, at the time of installation, the hospital had been denied a certificate of need, a new MRI unit was installed in a particular hospital with no immediate prospects of patient care reimbursement. The primary reason was that hospital administration believed that MRI represented a service that was critical for a tertiary hospital to provide. (There was also a belief that the certificate-of-need denial would eventually be reversed, which indeed did take place.)

8. *Outpatient Cardiac Catheterization Unit*. Although it would be more profitable to treat cardiac cath patients on an inpatient basis, the decision was made to introduce outpatient service primarily because the limited cardiology beds could then be used to treat more severely ill patients.

9. *Home Healthcare Investment*. The hospital joined a publicly funded for-profit company in the establishment of a firm that provides infusion therapies and related services to patients in their homes. One motivation was to reduce length of stay by enabling patients to receive treatment at home. Another important motivation was to derive a source of revenue from the joint venture that could support aspects of the tertiary hospitals' mission such as research and teaching that were not fully reimbursed.

10. *Investment in Software Development*. The hospital has made very significant investments in developing a management-control system that provides financial information to clinicians regarding the economic consequences of their decisions. The purpose of the investment was to improve the cost effectiveness of care provided in the hospital. Subsequently, the hospital created a for-profit subsidiary that has sold software to 100 hospitals throughout the country. The primary motivation of the investment was, again, to derive a return from investment that could support the tertiary hospital.

One might conclude from these 10 examples that these hospitals will soon go bankrupt because most of these investments will result in significant short-run losses in the hope that benefits will result in the long run. On the other hand, these examples illustrate that the decisions made at these hospitals did not involve just short-range financial issues, or quality issues, or marketing issues, or physician gratification issues. Instead they involve a complex set of judgments regarding how all of these criteria affected the institution. The central focus was to adopt strategies that addressed both short- and long-range goals of the institution. Particular attention was devoted in most cases to increasing inpatient activity with little direct concern for short-term financial consequences.

As to the future, while hospitals will continue to make significant investments in diagnostic and therapeutic technologies, they will invest more of their resources in technology that provides meaningful information. In the past, most investments in information have not had the financial or programmatic benefit that their promoters promised. Instead, hospitals have primarily automated clerical functions. Recent changes in technology offer the potential to use information to affect radically all forms of work performed within hospitals. Examples of new tools include bedside and hand-held terminals that include clinical-care plans as well as automated medical record systems that enable clinicians throughout the delivery system to have access to a patient's chart and that include extensive tools to aid in clinical decision-making and evaluation of outcome.

In conclusion, I am not particularly concerned that DRGs or competition will hinder the introduction of medical technology. The primary immediate concern of hospitals is to fill beds and ensure adequate payment. Few hospitals are actively making decisions that affect medical decision-making except in regard to PRO admission rules or length of stay. Moreover, regardless of the payment system, and even if capital is included in the DRG base, short-term financial considerations will never be the sole or even the primary criterion used in evaluating investments in medical technology. Instead, decision-making will continue to be based upon the integration of a number of factors including financial issues, marketing concerns, quality-of-care issues, and physician gratification.

As we move towards a more competitive delivery system, it is important to reflect that the ultimate consumer is not a PPO or a corporate benefits officer, but rather an individual patient. Patients, unlike payers, are concerned about quality, effectiveness, well being, and—to some extent—cost. Since patients are ultimately less concerned with cost than with effectiveness and amenities, hospital decision-making regarding the application of new technology will probably never be based upon short-range cost/benefit analyses affected by unit-of-payment formulae. Future decision-making regarding the application of technology will be primarily affected by strategic and programmatic criteria. It seems to me that this is the appropriate focus that best serves public policy.

8

The Myth of Reimbursement-Controlled Purchasing in Hospitals

Victor L. Rosenberg

One of the major factors altering the medical industry today is the continual emergence of new technologies and procedures. This, in itself, is not unique to health care, but in other industries there is more formal theory to explain how new ideas are evaluated and adopted. A six-month study of Massachusetts general care hospitals in 1986–1987 attempted to fill this void and to provide preliminary structure to our understanding of this issue.

A motivating factor in undertaking this study was the change under Medicare to the Prospective Payment System (PPS). It was anticipated that this change in the external environment of the hospital would influence the decision-making process for the adoption and utilization of new technology. PPS was expected to encourage the adoption of cost-reducing technology by providing hospitals with an incentive for assessing the impact of the cost of inpatient care on their financial position. However, determining how the PPS influenced the process of evaluating and adopting new ideas required a better understanding of the basic operation of this process within the health care industry.

The health care industry relies on a few simple myths about this process. Existing health care literature is full of these myths that have little or no data to support them, and major policy decisions are undertaken based on them.

Policymakers are aware of this lack of knowledge (Office of Technology Assessment, 1985), but researchers have developed justifications for acting on the myths, including: there is no research on what drives innovation in health care, and therefore we must use models that work in more traditional business settings (Roberts, 1982); hospital decision processes can be imputed by logic (Califano, 1986; Fein, 1986) although this path leads to divergent opinions about how the process "logically" works; and, hospital actions bear no relation to how other organizations act because the people are so different that there is no common reference (Weisbord, 1976).

I support a position expressed by Rosengren (1980) that there is an abundance of research; however, it lacks any organization into a workable theoretical description. The field has been well studied and poorly described.

This chapter builds on existing information about the behavior of health care organizations, and through systems-analysis methodology, selects the most critical mission information and addresses it through primary research.

The project was concerned with the promotion of effective technology. Since the effectiveness of an innovation can be evaluated only against some "goal," the research focused only on those situations where a clear goal existed, and where the hospital, when studied, was already considering alternative ways to apply its resources. This process is herein referred to as "tactical innovation." For operational purposes, tactical innovation includes finding new ways to use one's resources in meeting recognized goals and excludes serendipitous innovation, or innovation in marketing strategies.

The study examined how and why hospital managers support tactical innovation by promoting innovative alternatives to their current procedures. The results are based on focused interviews with 32 nonphysician directors of functional departments in 11 Massachusetts hospitals. These functional directors were asked to describe situations where tactical innovation was considered. They were first asked to describe the actual process that took place, including who was involved, what questions were asked, and what the sponsor received in reward or penalty. Then they were asked how they felt about the process, and would they support a similar project. Their responses were validated through interviews with hospital suppliers and group vice-presidents of hospital-management companies.

The hospital respondents represented the following departments: fiscal and reimbursement; material management; information services; marketing; nursing; pharmacy; laboratory; utilization review; and quality assurance.

Of note here is that as different as each department's tasks and concerns are, from business operations to actual patient care, respondents' answers to specific questions relative to tactical innovation were amazingly alike.

In all cases the major data in this study represent at least a 75% consensus among respondents. Overall, each respondent's answers were validated against another respondent at his or her site.

From these interviews a model was developed representing the process by which tactical innovation is sponsored. The model included:

• the steps in the process;
• the major obstacles to innovation; and
• the major management incentives promoting innovation.

This model is simple and easy to understand, yet it differs significantly from the two common myths about how hospitals operate.

The first common myth is that hospitals are independent entities with the ability to run themselves with self-determination, in a direct, simple, and predictable manner. It is rationalized then, that in changing their resources (controlled reimbursement dollars), they will automatically minimize costs to maximize profits. The economist's position that the system of reimbursement is the single most important force in driving innovation is one of the most prevalent myths. The argument is that when reimbursement is not based on cost, the industry will choose innovation that reduces cost.

The study challenges this myth; it provides insight into the process of innovation adoption, demonstrating how new ideas are evaluated differently by various types of decision makers and how current reimbursement changes that reward volume are affecting these decisions.

Of the many factors that impact innovation, reimbursement policy is of special interest because government and society use reimbursement, with limited success, to try to drive effective tactical innovation—use of resources. However, reimbursement policy is not the sole force driving or limiting change in health care. Specifically, controlled reimbursement dollars do not necessarily drive new efforts to control hospital costs. It is critical to understand why this is so, particularly if we are to design effective policies for controlling hospital costs.

The second myth is that hospitals are public-service ventures, not businesses, and that their directive is solely humanitarian, not money oriented. The rationale then follows that controlled reimbursement dollars will distort a good system.

THE STEPS IN THE PROCESS

Our study shows very consistent behavior in the process followed when proposing and evaluating tactical innovation. It also reveals that recent reimbursement policy pressures drive a variety of different hospital reactions, depending on the position of personnel, within the same hospital. Three basic groups were identified, each with a specific interest, and in turn, a different reaction to reimbursement policy pressures.

The first group consists of purchasing agents, materials managers, and money managers, people whose job it is to make purchases. Their primary interest in the hospital environment is in costs, and specifically, in dollar effectiveness. This group has reacted to the new reimbursement policy pressure with an increased cost-consciousness. It is imperative, to them, that they "buy better," not necessarily a different product, just the same product less expensively.

The second group identified consists of the clinicians, whose primary interest is in patient care. Cost-consciousness is minimal in this group. That pressure is overridden by other policy considerations, such as legal restrictions and by personal incentives, which are outside of a single hospital's control. Current policy has been able, however, to pressure clinicians to avoid unnecessary admissions and reduce hospital stays.

The third group is top administrative people responsible for matching revenues to costs. Contrary to expectation, it is easier for these people to find new revenues than to lower costs. Often, costs are raised in attempts to find revenues.

It should not be a surprise to find such diverse reactions from a complex dynamic organization, responding to accelerating outside pressure. While the effect is complex, it is not random. By laying out the steps, we can strive better to predict the effects of future policies.

Hospitals are divided along strict functional lines. Each function has its own licensing/certification system, and each is usually managed by a director with a background in that particular function. These functional directors have control of the functional procedures, and are the only individuals who can sponsor tactical innovation. This does not mean that it is the director's job to innovate, nor does it mean that he or she has the authority or even the discretion to innovate. It simply means that no one else directs specific procedures, and therefore, no one else can effectively cause those procedures to change.

In a traditional business we would expect someone to have specific responsibility to investigate actively improvements in current procedures. Standard business practices suggest that employees are expected to submit ideas, point out cost savings, and make suggestions, and many companies offer employee incentive programs for just that purpose. The study clearly revealed that nothing similar exists in a hospital environment. In fact, there is a single level of personnel who even might consider making such proposals.

Once a functional director has proposed a new idea, the hospital organization must evaluate it. The goal of the initial evaluation is to clarify the reasons for the idea and ensure that there is a consensus among all affected parties as to its acceptability. This evaluation seldom involves formal quantitative projections and does not review alternatives. This is a peer evaluation, not a management evaluation. The test of this step is that the idea is acceptable, not that it is optimal or even beneficial.

The initial administrative evaluation follows flexible format. Any of the following procedures is possible:

• The sponsor may be asked to prepare a report.
• The sponsor may receive help from finance or purchasing.
• The sponsor may be referred to a committee (any of a number of standing committees— a products committee, standards committee, patient care committee, information services committee, or a special committee set up to deal specifically with the matter at hand).

Consensus and acceptability are the central themes. Functional directors do not like taking sole responsibility for these actions and, in some cases, clearly stated that any decision they made could potentially result in patient death. Some functional directors reiterated the power of the medical staff and the chance that they could be fired should their idea seriously annoy a doctor (Holoweiko, 1983). Any change, in the sponsor's minds, could annoy medical staff, and therefore, the sponsors always want to diffuse the focus of that annoyance by spreading responsibility over a wide group.

From organizational theory, we can hypothesize a second reason for the intense need for consensus—measuring success. In a system where there are few measurable criteria, people are promoted based on the confidence that others have in them (Marcson, 1962). Group support for one's actions demonstrates trust; earning trust equates with successfully doing something in the hospital environment that pleases the masses involved, and the circle is complete.

Hospitals reject the importance of formal quantitative analysis so popular in general industry and government. There is no confidence that these methods can cope with the massive uncertainties of reimbursement policies, census, and labor supply. These methods are designed to evaluate alternative plans, and there is no requirement for considering more than one alternative in the hospital process.

Once the functional director makes his or her proposal—a reflection of the personal goals of that director—it automatically becomes the only viable idea. No other ideas have a sponsor: One must remember here that acceptability, not optimality or value, is the limited goal of the review.

At this stage, reimbursement policy is only a slight consideration. A proposal's value is not what is being evaluated; its acceptability is. Functional directors are basically unfamiliar with reimbursement rules.

Many hospitals have invested in new cost-accounting systems and new reimbursement-planning positions, but not in efforts to educate unit directors in economic issues. In fact, finance respondents considered the unit directors' ignorance in these areas justified. The rules are complicated and changing, and the respondents themselves have difficulty comprehending how it relates to individual decisions. Another interpretation of this response is that finance personnel do not want functional directors to understand the issues they were hired to understand.

In the sponsorship process, the physician's acceptance is critical for approval of any idea. While most hospitals, especially those with low census ratios, related that there was no formal participation by the physicians in the review process, all agreed that physicians, in the end, have an effective veto power. This fact is a constant frustration to the functional directors, who feel the physicians are not working with them. It lends impetus to the feeling among these directors that they do not have the discretionary power to work towards their own goals.

Functional directors feel that physicians avoid formal participation because they do not need to negotiate their issues. Physicians see themselves as customers of the hospital with the ability to leave at any time, taking their patients and revenues with them. Since revenue is a higher priority than profit (see Van Etten,

Chap. 7 of this volume), none felt that an individual functional director could risk losing even one physician's business. Thus, physicians' acceptance of a proposed idea is imperative for success.

At some point, the confusing issue of the physician's role in the resource allocation of general hospitals will have to be the subject of a study if we are to model successfully the resource planning of hospitals. The issue of importance to this study is not that physicians are an organizational problem but that they are perceived as such by the functional directors.

The personal goals, pressures, and incentives of functional directors and physicians differ. This creates conflict. The few hospitals found to be addressing the physician/power/participation issue demonstrated a more positive attitude towards innovation. Even at these sites strong skepticism remained about how fully the physicians embraced the hospital goals. Nonetheless, small demonstrations of cooperation proved highly effective.

The next step in the process of sponsoring tactical innovation is resource allocation. The initial evaluation only decided the acceptability of an idea, with no guarantee that the idea would get enough priority to receive resources. There is a budget process, usually an annual cycle, when all acceptable ideas are submitted for prioritization and resource allocation. Although allowance is made for some funding outside of this cycle, whenever possible, acceptable ideas are held and presented during the annual budget process. A few proposals, usually marketing ideas or crisis responses, are approved on their own value.

During the budget cycle the unit directors propose a prioritized list of their acceptable and supported proposals. These are often consolidated, by consensus, at a group meeting of senior management. On occasion, the CEO or finance department may make a first pass at the consolidation. As with the initial evaluation, the medical staff may comment independently and can contest the approved budget with the board.

Prioritization of proposals was the most consistent response to any interview question, and not at all what one would expect in a more traditional business orientation. Hospitals prioritize as follows: needs and imperatives are first, followed by revenue, and finally cost savings.

The existence of a class of imperative items is an alien concept to many business executives. In a traditional environment there are a number of expenses that could be considered imperative, but the American business ethic nonetheless requires them to be constantly questioned. In the hospital environment, the concept of imperatives may be basic to patient care or it may stem from a history of hospital costs being subsidized by society. Whatever the reason, and none of those interviewed could explain it or understand why I did not innately accept it, these imperatives are carved in stone. This may be the most significant area where a businessperson and a hospital manager cannot comprehend each other's stance.

Imperatives, proposals based on need, are given first priority. These include items needed for certification, equipment replacement, or support of a department falling behind in its workload.

Second priority goes to items that bring in revenues. Outpatient or nonhospital revenue, as generated from office buildings or home care for example, is most desirable, then revenues from high-profit inpatient product lines. Proposals that save money are given lowest priority in this process.

The interest in revenue-producing marketing issues over cost savings and even over profit is not unique. Other industries also value revenue over saving money since a successful revenue-generating project may produce more than expected and, more importantly, can open doors for future projects.

From a business standpoint, two issues are particularly peculiar. One is the credibility of marketing projections versus cost projections. Analysis of new revenue projects is minimal, usually based on logic. No respondents felt that they could prove marketing projections, so it was useless to try. But following the same logic pattern, none believes it possible to save money, so this was useless to try, as well! A very strong implication here is that this population wants to believe marketing projections and does not want to believe cost projections.

The other issue is that reducing costs is never seen as a marketing advantage. Lower costs do not lead to higher revenues as they do in other industries. This relationship between costs and revenues relies on two factors basic to understanding hospital economics. One, hospitals have constraints on capacity, and two, hospitals cannot compete on price. For these reasons lower costs cannot drive higher unit sales.

Traditional industry believes that the size of a market and the organizations that serve it are controlled by demand. If sufficient demand can be found or created, growth can occur quickly to meet it. In a hospital, however, the number of beds is fixed by physical plan and regulation. If more demand is found, the hospital must wade through a long process of approvals to build more beds.

In a traditional industry, the organization is always interested in reducing the price of services. This allows more effective competition, thereby increasing demand for products or services. A hospital must compete in areas other than price. Price is usually controlled by insurance companies or governments who decide, as payers, how much to allow for reimbursement of specific services.

Organizations in traditional industries have more to gain from cost reductions than do hospitals. These organizations see increased profits since lower costs raise margins; they also receive increased revenues because lower costs improve their competitive position, and they can expand to meet the increased demand. Hospitals, on the other hand, get only the first of these—higher margins.

The steps in the process of sponsoring tactical innovation, evaluation, resource allocation, and implementation are long and cumbersome. There appears to be no pressure to reach a timely response. For example, one vendor's market research revealed that hospital selection committees were content with two-year evaluations of software systems. Another example is that operational management positions, vice-presidents and directors, are often open for six-month executive searches.

Despite the slow process, fiscal people, like staff people everywhere, are concerned that decisions are made too fast, before finance has supplied its review and feedback. Financial analysis is unimportant in this environment. Finance is often asked to evaluate only how the proposal affects the finance department, e.g., whether it is billable, not whether it is good or bad.

THE MAJOR OBSTACLES TO INNOVATION

This definition of the process of sponsoring tactical innovation is required background, but does not address what drives the process—the incentives and disincentives. It is like defining the rules of a game; the outcome still cannot be predicted unless we know more about the players' internal and external motivations.

Within the hospital there is little direct, positive incentive for functional directors to be innovative. When they were asked the question, ''What do you receive for successfully implementing an innovation that helps the hospital?'' the standard response was ''Nothing.'' The most positive response was ''Professional satisfaction,'' an indirect incentive not under the control of the individual hospital.

A few sites do have bonus opportunities of up to $2,000 per year for exceptional work, a very small and temporary reward. Occasional small bonus plans do not make an attractive incentive program, especially with the high risks a functional director takes in sponsoring an innovation.

Hospitals have annual salary increases, but it is unclear that performance is a major criterion for salary growth. If general performance is not important, then effective use of resources is even less important. Annual increases are restricted to a narrow range, and total salary is limited based on job category and industry comparables. In addition, promotional opportunities are believed to be virtually nonexistent within the same hospital since hiring is based on functional qualifications, not past performance.

Functional directors are already at the ceiling of their career within the institution; they are heads of their professional areas of expertise within the hospital with no place to grow. While some functional directors are actually given areas of responsibility outside their own traditional areas, this is not perceived overall to be attainable. Even superior functional directors would need to return to school for an administrative degree to be considered for administration.

Good performance does not equal reward, nor does poor performance involve risk. Functional directors feel secure in their positions as department heads. Their position within the organization is at risk only if through change/innovation sponsorship they create an obvious conflict with the medical staff and/or risk an innovative attempt that leads to patient mortality; or, their department experiences chronic short-term production problems that lead to staff dissension.

Overall, in seeking incentives for growth, the functional director looks outside the present environment, which strangely enough, provides a direct incentive for performance to the maximum within the present organization.

Outside opportunities do exist at higher-paying, perhaps larger or more-specialized facilities, and these opportunities are based on one's professional achievements as recognized by others in the health care industry. Professional achievements do not necessarily mean meeting hospital manifest goals and do not lend themselves to growth within one's present environment. Building personal status is the growth key. One way to accomplish this includes finding reasons to present one's ideas and accomplishments at professional (health care industry) public meetings.

With these incentives, we expect and find the following operative goals for functional directors:

- maintaining harmony with the medical staff;
- promoting ideas for positive publicity within the profession;
- keeping one's staff satisfied; and
- delivering a certain level of production within the hospital.

Performance evaluation also enters into the incentive picture, and in turn is reflected in the individual's goals for sponsoring tactical innovation. Most respondents never mentioned hospital administration as a source of performance evaluation or feedback. Depending on their discipline, they mentioned physicians, peers, patients, and patients' families as their most common sources of performance evaluation, and this is reflected in their proposals. It must be remembered that they are at risk if the feedback is negative.

For example, nurses make recommendations for new beds that will directly benefit the patients. After all, the patients are directly tied to the nurse and nursing care. Lab directors make recommendations for faster test equipment that benefits the physician since the lab will hear directly from the physician if the work is faulty or they are seemingly unresponsive to a physician's request.

The farther away a department is from the physicians and patients, the more responsive it can be to hospital management without being at risk. Finance, for example, can implement new automated billing methods resulting in reduced staff, which would please hospital administrators concerned with meeting costs.

With insight into how departments and functional directors are affected when they sponsor innovation, we can certainly understand why it is done in such a peculiar manner. To a traditional American business executive, it is shocking. Capitalism exists on the premise of incentives. Good managers are an important resource and are kept by offering unlimited career options. They move from function to function within an organization, without regard for credentials. In traditional businesses, executives replace managers who are only coasting with managers who understand and support company policy.

The Medicare Prospective Payment System is supposed to provide incentives for efficient operation. Yet, in hospitals, the people responsible for deploying resources receive no incentive to conserve. The question then is: Do functional directors conserve anyway? The overall finding is no. Conserving to conserve in no way benefits functional directors, unless their positioning is removed from patient care and physician responsibility so that administration is their closest tie.

The rationale here is simple. Staff size directly reflects on the director's professional credentials and status and can be used as a positive point in moving to another facility at a higher salary. Knowing this, why would a functional director reduce staff even though open positions have not been filled and the staff has been operating satisfactorily?

Without any tangible reasons to manage resources effectively, functional directors do not see doing so as an objective. It is not, presently, a criterion for success; it is not measured.

The present process then, as we have come to find it, seems to promote two major obstacles to tactical innovation. First, there exists a lack of incentives for functional directors to support innovation; second, there exists a major risk in supporting anything that may annoy even a small segment of the medical staff.

Some hospitals address these obstacles better than others, but the problems remain the same. Let us look at the two obstacles more closely. Specifically, hospitals depend on functional directors to propose and implement change even though these people have minimal career expectations and see little reward for contributing to hospital goals. While we see evidence of increasing career opportunities for professionals, the new positions affect lower managers, not the functional directors themselves. Even for lower managers, these developing opportunities do not seem to have credibility to effect their goals.

Corporations that own or manage multiple hospitals offer expanded career options to innovative middle managers in many forms, and all hospitals encourage functional directors to create nonhospital services. Nonetheless, these do not seem to create significant incentives since they are viewed as exceptions and not as real opportunities towards which people can work. Employees and functional directors do not believe that management has an interest in their personal careers, and the validation interviews with senior management indicate that they are correct. When a management position opens up in a hospital, an outside search is conducted. Internal people are at a disadvantage.

Regarding the second obstacle, i.e., the risk in supporting anything that annoys any medical staff, functional directors exist in a precarious relationship to the medical staff. Physicians have a veto power over most procedures without having to accept any responsibility. Overall, functional directors must contend with the medical staff's power to overrule any proposal. Should a functional director gather support for a proposal that, in the end, annoys or inconveniences the medical staff, his or her job is in jeopardy, regardless of the proposal's merits.

Hospitals with high prestige and high census ratios did show significantly more interest in the difficult task of controlling medical staff loyalty and demonstrating the appearance of physician commitment to hospital goals. These hospitals exhibited the most innovative approaches to cost control. It appears, however, that the spirit of cooperation is a recent phenomenon since the advent of cost containment.

It is interesting to note also that the hospitals in this category exhibited the appearance more than the reality of cooperation. Individual directors still cited personal goals as more important than hospital goals. Yet these same directors seemed more comfortable and secure in suggesting innovations.

On the surface, it would appear that these weak incentives and overwhelming disincentives to innovation would be counterproductive to hospital profitability. To understand why these actually support the present hospital system, we must look to the hospital's economic incentives.

We have been led to believe that the new reimbursement controls (e.g., the Medicare Prospective Payment System, utilization review, case management, preferred provider organizations, prepaid health plans, and health maintenance organizations, among others) will push hospitals to lower their cost structures. We know from the study that this is not necessarily so. The key to understanding the real hospital economic goals lies in two previously noted observations:

• there is increasing interest in marketing the hospital to physicians; and,
• there is a different relationship between hospital and physician in those hospitals with high utilization, which leads to improved attitudes towards cost containment.

From the interviews with senior hospital management, a curious model of their incentives emerged. Cost containment is creating a debilitating overcapacity and lowering total hospital utilization by rejecting "unnecessary" services. Some observers call this less care, not less-expensive care.

Despite overcapacity, hospitals have many good business reasons for not closing down their beds even if they are chronically empty. Hospitals see their costs as fixed and do not perceive a cost advantage in closing down services. This view of costs may or may not be accurate, but it is the hospital view. Also, hospital beds are licensed, and if the hospital closes one down, it may not receive permission for reinstatement. Hospitals differ from most industries in that they are of a relatively fixed size; they cannot easily or arbitrarily expand.

Hospitals cannot compete on pricing; as noted earlier, they do not control their prices. The government and insurers decide what is an "equitable reimbursement" and pay the hospital accordingly. The only basis by which some reimbursement plans differentiate among hospitals is on historical costs or prevailing local rates. Neither of these provides room for competition.

With the pressures of overcapacity, low marginal cost, high exit costs, and inability to control price, hospitals must solicit revenue by providing attractive services to the physician. These take several forms: social service (prestige); physical service (easy admissions); and direct service (stipend or salary guarantee).

Understanding that there are two classes of hospitals, those with high prestige and those without, we can comprehend why high-prestige hospitals are more able to keep their beds full. Their prestige attracts physicians. They can afford to push for cost improvements, which may offend some physicians, because they have others waiting to use their services. The rest of the hospitals need to accept increased costs in order to attract physicians. For most hospitals the financial need to attract adequate revenues outweighs the financial need to reduce costs.

This leads to a clear set of hospital operative goals:

1. Concentrate expenses on better market position to fill capacity and only pursue cost savings when the hospital reaches capacity.
2. Avoid any action that may offend physicians, unless it is a high-prestige hospital that can experiment with cost reductions and/or physician discipline.
3. Pursue ways to diversify or control the product mix. All hospitals look for non-inpatient revenue.
4. Save money in ways that cannot hurt competitive position. This allows hospitals to search for the best way to purchase an item once the item has become generic. Material management can be cost conscious without upsetting the physicians.

This odd economic system also supports the most puzzling of the study findings. The career system seems to prefer that a functional director put his or her best efforts into finding an outside job!

As noted earlier, the director finds the next job by investing personal effort into promoting a public image within the industry. In doing so, the hospital also is promoted. This adds to the hospital's prestige and helps attract critical revenue.

The study clearly reveals that none of the circulating theories relative to how hospitals allocate resources is 100% correct or 100% wrong. What we have found is a confusing blend of personal prestige, institutional goals, professional goals, disincentives that translate into personal incentives, and incentives that are individually sponsored rather than organizationally developed and sponsored, all functioning independently while being dependent on the host organization.

Overall, despite what traditional business executives might call peculiar incentives and overwhelming disincentives in the process of sponsoring tactical innovation, the present hospital system works. Cost containment has not necessarily had much impact on the operative goals of this process (see Van Etten, Chap. 7 of this volume) but we can see an impact on the process.

- There is improvement in how traditional commodities are purchased. Better prices are being negotiated.
- There is an interest in strategic planning. Hospitals are finding new business opportunities.
- There is pressure to justify expenses. However, less formal project analysis is being done.

Does this imply that no change in public policy can impact this complex system? Absolutely not.

The study implies that it is possible to bring together much of the existing knowledge about hospital organizations and related environmental pressures to construct a rational model of how the system operates. Through targeted research we can test and redefine this model until it is internally consistent and shows an understandable response to fixed environmental factors, thus providing avenues for change.

9

Technological and Cost Implications of Changing Hospital Staffing Patterns

Henry P. Brehm and Sally Brewster Moulton

Major increases in the cost of inpatient hospital care and in staff-to-patient ratios have occurred in U.S. hospitals since the early 1960s (American Hospital Association, 1987). Over the same period hospitals adopted a wide array of expensive new technologies. The literature is explicit concerning the important role of these new medical technologies in the growth of hospital costs (Feldstein, 1981; Goldfarb et al., 1980). While the substantial increase in the proportion of staff to patients undoubtedly also has been a significant factor in the growing cost of inpatient care, published research barely examines this issue (Barocci, 1981, 101; Shapleigh, 1985). These ratio changes have been noted (Feldstein, 1981; Goldfarb et al., 1980) but not made the focus of analysis, possibly because such data are not used in hospital planning. However, the significance for rising hospital costs of rising staff-to-patient ratios should be recognized as a factor in its own right. Increases in these ratios have an impact on costs separate from those of new technology and growth in earnings per employee.

The relationship between trends in staffing patterns, technology utilization, and costs is the focus of this chapter. We discuss the growth in staff-to-patient ratios in the context of changing technology utilization and rising inpatient care costs. We also consider the impacts on hospital staffing and technology adoption decisions of the increasingly cost-conscious environment in which hospitals now operate. Relevant policy issues that health planners must consider are identified in the concluding section.

THEORETICAL PERSPECTIVE

The interplay among trends in hospital staffing, technology, and costs is analyzed from a sociology of organizations point of view, using open systems and organization-as-process perspectives. Open systems theory states that an organization interacts with its external environment. There is an ongoing exchange between them, with the organization obtaining inputs from the environment and providing outputs to it in return. The nature of this exchange is crucial to organizational well-being. It also shapes the internal structure of organizations, and this is of particular relevance to our discussion of hospital staffing patterns (Hall, 1972, 23–25). Organizations and their components vary in the extent to which they depend upon, and are therefore vulnerable to pressures from, the different elements of their environments (Hall, 1982, 236; Jacobs, 1974). Furthermore, because both organizations and environments change over time, the relationship between them is intrinsically dynamic.

The organization-as-process perspective focuses on "all activities necessary for delineating organizational goals, assembling human and other resources, structuring work and authority relationships, establishing communication channels, and adapting organizational responses to internal and external demands. This process builds the entity called an organization and then continues to modify organization structure." An organization usually tries to adapt to its environment in order to be successful, with the result that organizational structure is in a continuous state of flux (Levey & Loomba, 1984, 150).

These two perspectives help analyze the nature and implications of hospital-environment interaction over the last several decades by illuminating the impact of environmental factors on organizational decision-making in areas such as hospital staffing and use of technology. The next section describes environmental factors that exerted significant influences on these types of decisions.

HISTORY OF ENVIRONMENTAL CHANGES AFFECTING THE HOSPITAL INDUSTRY

The National Hospital Survey and Construction Act of 1946 (the Hill-Burton Act) established a funding mechanism for the development of additional hospital bed capacity in the United States (Raffel, 1984). The motivation for this program no doubt lay in the nation's emergence from the 1930s depression and World War II with pent-up demand for increased availability of hospital space. In the postwar environment, which frankly encouraged the growth of hospital capacity, insurers ranging from Blue Cross to Medicare developed a health insurance model that emphasized reimbursement for hospitalization in order to reduce the damaging financial impact of hospital costs on the individual (Brehm & Coe, 1980). Retrospective cost reimbursement by third-party payers became the standard form of payment (Langwell & Moore, 1982), and by the mid–1980s, private and government insurers were paying for roughly 90% of hospital care (Kahl &

Clark, 1986). On the positive side, this financing mechanism made hospital care affordable for a much greater percentage of the population. However, by virtue of the fact that it paid for practically all costs, third-party insurance also insulated providers and users from the impacts of rising costs, at least for a time (Kahl & Clark, 1986).

So long as it was taken for granted that third-party payers would cover the costs of whatever care was provided and a not-for-profit orientation predominated, the quality rather than the cost of care could be, and was, the chief focus in the hospital industry. Benefit to health was measured in terms of the ability to provide the highest available quality of care to the patient (Langwell & Moore, 1982). Benefit relative to cost, including careful review of actual organizational need based on such factors as patients served does not seem to have been a primary concern (Kahl & Clark, 1986) in either the consideration and adoption of new technology (Barocci, 1981, 89, 91) or the employment of additional staff. Furthermore, costs were recoverable so long as there was some minimum level of use in a facility.

Since these circumstances made new technology relatively easy to justify and finance, one way that hospitals improved the quality of care was by continually upgrading the type and range of services offered. At best, then, there were limited incentives to control costs and strong incentives to add staff and the latest technology and care modalities, so long as there was a perceived benefit to health. Such an environment almost certainly fostered more expansion in each of these areas than would have occurred had cost/benefit analyses been an important factor in decision-making. This situation greatly contributed to the escalating costs that have become a hallmark of the industry.

As hospital costs surged out of control in the 1970s and early 1980s, a variety of interest groups began to press for utilization review, cost reduction, and increased efficiency. In particular, employers, third-party payers, and consumers sought ways of controlling the rising costs of inpatient care.

Gradually, a variety of cost-control mechanisms came into being. Hospital certificate-of-need (CON) requirements were introduced in the 1970s to control the increase of bed capacity, the duplication of resources, and the diffusion of new technology. The point had been reached where the incentives offered by the Hill-Burton Act were no longer appropriate. Professional standards review organizations (PSROs), also introduced in the 1970s, were intended to control the use of inpatient care under Medicare (PSROs were later replaced by peer review organizations). In 1983, Medicare initiated its Prospective Payment System (PPS), a revolutionary move aimed at standardizing payments to hospitals for inpatient care.

Under the PPS, Medicare reimburses hospitals based on the average cost associated with each of 467 diagnosis-related groups (DRGs), and not on the cost of care actually provided to each patient. In practice, hospitals recover more than they have spent for some patients and less than they have spent on others. The resulting incentive is obvious: the organization's economic well-being requires maximizing the former situation and minimizing the latter. Using only this economic guideline, however, could result in significantly underserving certain segments of the population, e.g., those within a DRG who require more than average health care services.

By fixing the amount of reimbursement that hospitals receive per patient for specific diagnoses, Medicare has obtained potentially greater control over its expenditures. Because of this anticipated advantage and also because Medicare patients represent a large and growing segment of the population served by many hospitals, it is likely that other third-party payers will adopt a similar approach (Appelbaum & Granrose, 1986; Coddington, Palmquist & Trollinger, 1985; Crawford & Fottler, 1985).

The prospective payment mechanism means that hospitals must exert new and greater controls over the use of their resources in the treatment of each patient. At the same time, as will be discussed in a later section, reduced admissions since 1982 have increased the competition for patients. Another significant factor in the growth of competition since the 1970s has been the growth in the numbers and economic importance of for-profit hospitals. From 1972 to 1986, for-profit hospital beds more than doubled as a percentage of total hospital beds in the United States (3.7% to 8.3%) (American Hospital Association, 1987, Table 1). This forced the not-for-profit segment of the industry, still by far the dominant segment, to reorient itself accordingly. The onset of aggressive competition not only required hospitals to devote resources to maintaining or increasing their market share but also to pay more attention to the efficiency of their operations, the appropriate use of services and resources, and the costs of care delivered. Long-established values demanding the provision of high-quality care combined with the Medicare reimbursement change and the increasingly competitive health care market, have presented hospitals with contradictory pressures that they must reconcile in order to function effectively.

TRENDS IN HOSPITAL STAFFING

In general, little information has been available concerning longitudinal changes in the hospital industry's occupational structure (Barocci, 1981) except for a few data series from the American Hospital Association. Perhaps, as already noted, this was the result of hospital management criteria that typically have not required the development of data bases pertinent to the control of resources, including personnel (Shapleigh, 1985). Some recent studies as well as emerging hospital data collection efforts have begun to address the gap (Applebaum & Granrose, 1986; Kahl & Clark, 1986; Kotelchuck, 1986).

Growth in Total Hospital Employment

Hospital employment increased 134% from 1960 to its peak in 1982, or from 1,598,000 to 3,746,000 full-time equivalent (FTE) personnel. It then fell slightly (about 3%) from 1983 to 1985 (see Table 9.1). This decline in the 1980s was

Table 9.1
Characteristics of Total U.S. Hospitals[1]

Year	Admissions*	Beds*	Average Daily Census*	FTE personnel Number*	Per 100 Census**
1960	25,027	1,658	1,402	1,598	114
1965	28,812	1,704	1,403	1,952	139
1970	31,759	1,616	1,298	2,537	195
1971	32,664	1,556	1,237	2,589	209
1972	33,265	1,550	1,209	2,671	216
1973	34,352	1,535	1,189	2,769	233
1974	35,506	1,513	1,167	2,919	250
1975	36,157	1,466	1,125	3,023	269
1976	36,776	1,434	1,090	3,108	285
1977	37,060	1,407	1,066	3,213	301
1978	37,243	1,381	1,042	3,280	315
1979	37,802	1,372	1,043	3,382	324
1980	38,892	1,365	1,060	3,492	329
1981	39,169	1,362	1,061	3,661	345
1982	39,095	1,360	1,053	3,746	356
1983	38,887	1,350	1,028	3,707	361
1984	37,938	1,339	970	3,630	374
1985	36,304	1,318	910	3,625	398
1986	35,219	1,290	883	3,647	413

Change In Item Over 5-Year Intervals (in percents)

1960-65	15		0	22	22
1965-70	10		-7	30	40
1970-75	14		-13	19	38
1975-80	8		-6	16	22
1980-85	-7		-14	4	21

[1]Figures taken from American Hospital Association, 1987, Table 1 Trends in Utilization, Personnel and Finances for Selected years 1946 through 1986.

*In thousands.

**This figure calculated using unadjusted average daily census.

the first since the collection of hospital employment data began in 1946. The biggest percentage increases occurred in the 1960s, which saw a 22% rise from 1960 to 1965 and a 30% rise from 1965 to 1970. Although the rate of growth slowed in the 1970s, hospital employment continued to increase substantially in terms of absolute numbers. In sharp contrast, it grew just 4% from 1980 to 1986, including the 1983–85 decline. As will be seen in the following sections, the enormous overall growth in hospital personnel from 1960 to 1986 was not associated with similar rates of growth in hospital utilization, e.g., admissions and average daily census.

Growth in Staff-to-Patient Ratio

The ratio of FTE hospital personnel per 100 patients showed a very substantial increase nationally for all types of hospitals from 1960 to 1986 (see Table 9.1).[1]

For all U.S. hospitals it grew by 362%, rising continuously from 114 FTE personnel per 100 patients in 1960 to 413 per 100 in 1986 (see Table 9.1).[2] Although the fastest growth occurred from 1965 to 1975, the rate of increase was never less than 20% in any five-year interval after 1960. This pattern is evident regardless of whether one uses average daily census data that are unadjusted (since 1960) or adjusted (since 1965). It is well worth noting that the growth rate in the staff-to-patient ratio did not slow after 1982. That is, its pattern of continuous growth did not change as an immediate result of either Medicare's Prospective Payment System introduced in 1983 or the declines in the absolute numbers of FTE personnel between 1983 and 1985.

The causes of the rapid growth in the staff-to-patient ratio need to be understood. A rising ratio may have been required to support significant ongoing improvements in the quality of care provided. Alternatively, it may have been associated with some (possibly considerable) degree of redundancy. In fact each explanation may be applicable, but to different areas of hospital operations. There are obvious implications for hospital management as well as for the provision of the desired quality of health care in the present cost-conscious era. Cutting the staff-to-patient ratio as a means of economizing is appropriate where unnecessary redundancy exists. However, some redundancy may be required during slack periods to ensure adequate coverage during peak utilization. In those cases where the proportion of staff to patients was deliberately increased in order to provide a particular type of care, reducing the ratio may threaten the hospital's ability to continue providing that care.

Changes in the Occupational Mix

The occupational composition of hospitals is another aspect of staffing trends that deserves close attention. It would make sense, especially as the staff-to-patient ratio has risen steadily, to investigate the extent to which each hospital occupation has shared in this growth. Presumably, differences do exist among the various occupations. However, it is not entirely clear at present where changes in the organizational and occupational structures led to increases in staff-to-patient ratios, and for what functional purpose.

The health occupations and professions that function within the hospital have limited upward mobility structures because of training and licensing requirements. Possibly this lack of opportunity has influenced hospital staffing patterns (Barocci, 1981, 171). We suggest that it may have led to an increased tendency to hire paraprofessionals and aides not only to provide needed help but also to elevate the social status of specific occupations and professions by increasing the number of levels below them. As cost containment and competition were not motivating factors for hospital organizational behavior until relatively recently, positional enhancement would have faced fewer constraints than in other settings or than may exist currently in the hospital setting.

Hospital managers have met recent needs for cost containment with various strategies (Egdahl & Walsh, 1985). Labor costs are a major target because they represent a high percentage of total hospital costs (Barocci, 1981, 111; Kahl & Clark, 1986). However, unlike some industries, the nature of health care services has not permitted the substitution of capital for labor (Aries & Kennedy, 1986). It has been argued that because of this, management is trying to cut labor costs by breaking tasks down into simpler components so they can be performed by lower-paid individuals, and by efforts to increase productivity as measured by procedures performed in a period of time. The presumption is that such strategies have resulted in the proliferation of low-paying jobs, reduced opportunity for advancement, and increased management-labor tensions (Aries & Kennedy, 1986). If this has indeed been the case, then cost-containment strategies may have resulted in changes in the occupational mix as well as increases in the staff-to-patient ratio.

Some tentative clues about recent trends in occupational mix can be gleaned from a study of the employment impacts of DRGs in a nonrandom sample of Philadelphia hospitals (Applebaum & Granrose, 1986). In these hospitals, the proportion of clerical to health care workers has increased as more clerical workers have been hired to cope with DRG-related administrative tasks. While some occupations related to inpatient care (e.g., food service) have declined, others, including some medical technician occupations, have grown slightly because of the introduction of new technology. Cutbacks have occurred in lower-skilled health care jobs (e.g., nurse's aides and licensed practical nurses), but registered nurse employment has remained stable. Administrators in this study apparently believe that a more highly skilled staff (i.e., of registered nurses) is more flexible and thus more cost effective. In the nursing area, then, deskilling has not been used as a cost-control method, contrary to the argument advanced in the previous paragraph. These findings cannot be used to create an overall picture of shifts in the distribution of hospital employment by occupation, even in the Philadelphia area. They do suggest, however, the types of changes that should be investigated in a more comprehensive study.

Other sources indicate that clerical workers have grown substantially as a percentage of the hospital labor force over the last two decades. However, in terms of absolute numbers, the growth of clinical support personnel (a subset of health care workers) has far outpaced that of the clerical group (Committee on Technology and Health Care, 1979; Aries & Kennedy, 1986).

Employment projections by the Bureau of Labor Statistics for 1984–95 assume that support occupations (e.g., clerical, cleaning, housekeeping, and protective service) will decline, while professional, managerial, and clinical jobs will rise as a proportion of the hospital labor force (Kahl & Clark, 1986). Lower-skilled occupations are expected to show slower-than-average growth for the industry. These projections lend some support to the Philadelphia study insofar as the nurse's aide and LPN occupations are expected to decline under the BLS's low-growth scenario in which hospitals slow the introduction of technology and face severe reimbursement restrictions and declining utilization (Kahl & Clark, 1986).

Hospital occupational mix will bear close watching into the future to assess the actual in contrast to the presumed impact of cost-containment efforts that are based on changes in utilization and reimbursement patterns.

EXPLAINING HOSPITAL STAFFING TRENDS

We would like to know what factors inside as well as outside the hospital contributed to the observed national trends in hospital employment and staffing ratios and just what role each played. There are two general categories of likely candidates: changes in the availability and utilization of hospitals, and changes in the nature of the health care services the hospital provides and how it functions in providing them. Items in the first category would be expected to affect hospital employment levels. However, unless they interacted with what the hospital did and/or how it did it, they logically should not influence staff-to-patient ratios. Changes in hospital availability and utilization relate to hospital admissions, average daily census, average length of stay, number of beds, and occupancy rate. Items in the second category (i.e., changes in the nature of health care services) could affect both employment levels and staff-to-patient ratios. This includes the use of health care technology, care intensity, and activities related to administrative requirements and the need to conform with a variety of regulations imposed by external agencies. Case mix is an intervening issue, potentially interacting with both categories of factors. Hospital strategy, which can affect and be affected by considerations within these general areas, is itself an issue of concern, especially since the environment in which hospitals function has undergone some very major changes in recent years.

The following sections discuss these issues, starting with hospital case mix because of its potential impact on other factors.

Case Mix

Case mix, i.e., the type and/or severity of cases treated, has changed over time for a variety of reasons. For example, over the last several decades, average life expectancy has been increasing, especially among the oldest segments of the population. Increased life expectancy for the elderly does not necessarily imply better health (Rice & Feldman, 1983). Those who live longer but in relatively poor health require more, and sometimes more intensive, care than earlier cohorts in which the sickest members generally died sooner. This, in combination with population aging, has already resulted in a greater proportion of geriatric hospital cases. Changes in case mix also have resulted from new treatment modalities that make is possible to treat more types of conditions on an outpatient basis, which obviously alters the composition of inpatient cases. As the case mix changes, the type of treatment and the labor intensity required may change as well. When this happens, a different occupational mix may also be needed. For this reason, one would expect to find that shifts in the distribution of hospital employment by occupation have occurred in recent decades.

Changes in Hospital Availability and Utilization

Total hospital admissions rose 57% from 1960 to 1981, or from 25 to 39 million, and then fell 10% from 1981 to 1986; the same pattern can be seen for short-term general hospitals that had 92% of all admissions in 1960 and in 1986 (see Tables 9.1 and 9.2). For all U.S. hospitals, the average daily census plateaued in the early 1960s at 1.4 million. Since then, it basically has fallen steadily so that in 1986 it was 883,000, a 37% decline from 1965.

The decline in average daily census was accounted for not by a change in utilization of short-term general hospitals but by a change in how nonfederal psychiatric hospitals function (see Tables 9.1–9.4). Annual admissions to these psychiatric hospitals grew to about 600,000 in the early 1970s and have remained fairly stable since then, as have occupancy rates. The number of beds in such hospitals peaked at 722,000 in 1960 and have been declining ever since, reaching 167,000 in 1986. Obviously, admissions to these hospitals have changed in nature. The same number of admissions now can be handled with a much smaller number of beds. Because of changes in treatment approach, patients have shorter lengths of stay than was previously the case. As a result, there has been a decline in the average daily census among nonfederal psychiatric hospitals, from 672,000 in 1960 to 143,000 in 1986, accounting for the entire decline seen in average daily census for all U.S. hospitals.

Nonfederal short-term general and other special hospitals[3] actually showed increases in average daily census through 1981, when it started to decline along with admissions. These data indicate that some portion of the increase in employment may have been related to an increase in admissions. However, the increases in employment far exceeded those in admissions and average daily census, producing the observed pattern of increases in staff-to-patient ratio.

The average length of stay in nonfederal short-term general hospitals was 8.2 days in 1970, moved down slowly to 7.6 days by 1977, and stayed at that level until 1984 when it started to decline again, reaching 7.1 days in 1986 (see Table 9.2). These declines occurred despite the trend toward an older and potentially sicker population. While this might seem paradoxical, a variety of new approaches to treatment make it possible to discharge hospital patients sooner. Another factor in length-of-stay trends is that, until recently, admission rates were rising (National Center for Health Statistics, 1980–1985). Rising admission rates sometimes relate to a drop in case severity and, therefore, shorter average lengths of stay. The observed combination of reduced average length of stay and increased admissions may not reflect a more serious case mix, but may nevertheless contribute to a higher staff-to-patient ratio because shorter hospital stays are more care intensive.

Occupancy rates for short-term hospitals ranged between a high of 78.0% and

Table 9.2
Characteristics of Nonfederal Short-Term General and Other Special Hospitals[1]

Year	Admissions*	Beds*	Adjusted Average Daily Census*	Average Length of Stay (days)	Occupancy Rate (%)	Outpatient Visits*	FTE personnel Number*	FTE personnel Per 100 Adjusted Census
1960	22,970	639	---	7.6	74.7	------	1,080	---
1965	26,463	741	620	7.8	76.0	92,631	1,386	224
1970	29,252	848	727	8.2	78.0	133,545	1,929	265
1971	30,142	867	736	8.0	76.7	148,423	1,999	272
1972	30,777	884	739	7.9	75.2	166,983	2,056	278
1973	31,761	903	768	7.8	75.4	178,939	2,149	280
1974	32,943	931	793	7.8	75.3	194,838	2,289	289
1975	33,519	947	806	7.7	74.8	196,311	2,399	298
1976	34,068	961	816	7.7	74.4	207,725	2,483	304
1977	34,353	974	820	7.6	73.6	204,238	2,581	315
1978	34,575	980	825	7.6	73.5	204,461	2,662	323
1979	35,160	988	841	7.6	73.8	203,873	2,762	328
1980	36,198	992	861	7.6	75.4	206,752	2,879	334
1981	36,494	1,007	876	7.6	75.9	206,729	3,039	347
1982	36,429	1,015	882	7.6	75.2	250,888	3,110	353
1983	36,201	1,021	869	7.6	73.4	213,995	3,102	357
1984	35,202	1,020	824	7.3	68.9	216,474	3,023	367
1985	33,501	1,003	780	7.1	64.8	222,773	3,003	385
1986	32,410	982	774	7.1	64.2	234,270	3,032	392

[1]Figures taken from American Hospital Association, 1987, Table 1 Trends in Utilization, Personnel and Finances for selected years 1946 through 1986.

*In thousands.

114

Table 9.3

Characteristics of Investor-Owned (For-Profit) Short-Term General and Other Special Hospitals[1]

Year	Admissions*	Beds*	Adjusted Average Daily Census*	Occupancy Rate (%)	FTE personnel Number*	FTE personnel Per 100 Adjusted Census
1960	1,550	37	--	65.4	48	--
1965	1,844	47	--	68.6	70	--
1970	2,031	53	41	72.2	97	238
1971	2,088	54	41	71.0	100	245
1972	2,161	57	42	68.7	105	249
1973	2,334	63	47	68.3	117	249
1974	2,553	70	52	67.5	133	257
1975	2,646	73	53	65.9	139	263
1976	2,734	76	54	64.8	147	272
1977	2,849	80	57	64.6	159	279
1978	2,880	81	57	63.8	165	290
1979	2,963	83	59	63.9	174	297
1980	3,165	87	62	65.2	189	304
1981	3,239	88	63	66.4	203	322
1982	3,316	91	66	65.5	212	320
1983	3,299	94	66	63.1	213	323
1984	3,314	100	64	57.0	214	334
1985	3,242	104	63	52.1	221	350
1986	3,231	107	65	50.7	229	354

[1]Figures taken from American Hospital Association, 1987, Table 1 Trends in Utilization, Personnel and Finances for Selected years 1946 through 1986.

*In thousands.

Table 9.4
Characteristics of Nonfederal Psychiatric Hospitals[1]

Year	Admissions*	Beds*	Average Daily Census*	Outpatient Visits*	FTE personnel Number*	Per 100 Census**
1960	362	722	672	-----	238	35
1965	491	685	607	1,003	274	45
1970	598	527	447	2,740	305	68
1971	602	469	393	2,988	285	72
1972	585	457	378	4,139	307	81
1973	588	422	342	4,611	303	89
1974	595	383	307	5,240	308	100
1975	604	330	265	5,287	292	110
1976	598	291	230	5,496	285	124
1977	587	261	211	5,018	287	136
1978	580	235	190	5,602	278	146
1979	567	224	187	5,614	282	151
1980	566	215	183	4,630	275	150
1981	558	202	174	4,976	275	158
1982	568	195	168	5,392	277	165
1983	552	185	160	5,713	264	165
1984	578	175	151	5,206	260	172
1985	602	171	147	4,902	263	179
1986	607	167	143	5,427	263	184

[1]Figures taken from American Hospital Association, 1987, Table 1 Trends in Utilization, Personnel and Finances for Selected years 1946 through 1986.

*In thousands.

**This figure calculated using unadjusted average daily census.

a low of 73.4% for the years from 1960 through 1983 (see Table 9.2), and then declined to 64.2% by 1986. This recent drop reflects the combined impact of reduced admissions and a lower average length of stay. The lower occupancy rate, since it can directly affect profitability and heighten interest in cutting costs, probably influenced the 1983–85 decrease in hospital employment.

The data also reflect the drop in admissions and daily census that started in the early 1980s and has contributed to industry competition. This decline was proportionately much greater than the 1983–85 drop in FTE employees. Consequently, the upward trend in the staff-to-patient ratio continued unabated through those years of decreasing employment.

Whether this upward trend was deliberate or unintended is not clear. For example, despite growing cost-consciousness, beliefs about the necessity of increasing the staff-to-patient ratio to provide specific types of care may have resulted in continued expansion. Alternatively, the staff-to-patient ratio may not have been perceived as an issue and, therefore, was not sufficiently visible to attract administrative attention and action; i.e., its growth was incidental. Other factors, such as the interests of various occupational bases of power within the hospital, may also have contributed to the growth in this ratio. These would include physicians' requirements for technical staff support availability and nursing standards for patient-load coverage.

There has been no major change in the number of hospitals in the United States since about 1965. The small changes that did occur related to a decline in long-term hospitals and an increase in nonfederal psychiatric ones. However, for number of beds the situation is different. The number of short-term hospital beds, except for those in for-profit hospitals, rose through 1983 and then started to decline, reflecting the more recent pattern of reduced use of inpatient care (see Table 9.2). By contrast, the number of beds in for-profit hospitals has increased steadily. Nevertheless, the total number of beds in all U.S. hospitals has fallen steadily since 1965 (see Table 9.1) because of a drop in long-term beds including those in psychiatric and federal hospitals. That short-term general hospital beds rose from 39% of all hospital beds in 1960 to 76% in 1986 pointedly indicates the decreased availability of long-term beds.

Despite the reductions in beds and average daily census, employment levels in long-term and federal hospitals did not decrease appreciably. This accounts in part for the overall increase in staff-to-patient ratio, although staffing ratios are much lower in long-term and federal hospitals than in short-term hospitals. These trends can be seen most clearly for nonfederal psychiatric hospitals (see Table 9.4), the largest category of long-term hospitals.

The unrelenting growth in staff-to-patient ratios has continued despite these recent changes in the availability and use of hospital services that might have been expected to reverse the trend. To this point, the discussion has focused only on the relationship between inpatient care and staffing, since the ratios are calculated using only the inpatient measure, average daily census. The question can be raised as to whether trends in outpatient care use also may have affected staffing ratios.

Outpatient visits per year to short-term hospitals slightly more than doubled between 1965 and 1976 (see Table 9.2). In the 10 years since then, outpatient visits have ranged from 200–250 million each year. Recent growth, however, is not sufficient to account for the increasing staff-to-patient ratio. Furthermore, the pattern of increased outpatient visits between 1965 and 1986 is not similar to that for the growth in the staffing ratio.

For nonfederal psychiatric hospitals, outpatient visits increased five-fold between 1965 and 1974, reaching over 5 million per year (see Table 9.4). They have been stable at that level ever since. Presumably, staff functions shifted to accommodate the heavier reliance on outpatient care as well as a changed approach to inpatient treatment. However, neither the FTE employment numbers nor the pattern of growth in staff-to-patient ratio match the pattern of outpatient visits even considering compensating declines in beds and average daily census. Overall, the increase in outpatient visits does not explain the increases in the staff-to-patient ratio.

Differences by Hospital Type

Variations can be seen by hospital type in the data on staffing patterns. These variations are important from a policy perspective since they affect not only the focus of management strategies but also which strategies will be effective for a given type of hospital. Furthermore, in order to interpret the overall hospital data correctly, it is necessary to know in which types of hospitals the source of change or continuity is located.

When FTE staff-to-patient ratios are examined by hospital type, it becomes clear that the trend seen for all U.S. hospitals combined is present also for each subgroup. Although growth was the industrywide pattern, the rate of growth varied substantially by segment. For example, from 1972 to 1986, the FTE staff-to-patient ratio grew by 42% in for-profit short-term hospitals and by 127% in nonfederal psychiatric hospitals (see Tables 9.3 and 9.4).

While the staff-to-patient ratio has risen in every type of hospital, the pattern of growth in absolute numbers of employees has been quite different across hospital types. Since 1972, the total number of FTE personnel has increased steadily in for-profit hospitals (see Table 9.3). In nonfederal psychiatric hospitals, it peaked in 1974 and has since fluctuated somewhat but declined overall by about 15% (see Table 9.4). This occurred along with the large increase in the staff-to-patient ratio based primarily on the change in inpatient numbers. These patterns for FTE personnel differ from the one for all hospitals reviewed earlier, where the peak was in 1982, employment fell through 1985, and increased again in 1986 (see Table 9.1).

Hospital Strategy

The choices hospitals make as they adapt to changes in their external environment potentially affect any and every aspect of their management and operations, including, of course, technology utilization and staffing patterns. Hospital management strategies are being developed to deal with a range of issues—competition, external regulation (e.g., CON requirements), cash reserve access, development, and endowment. Strategic moves include restructuring (introducing multihospital corporations, parent holding companies, and joint ventures), and refocusing of priorities (e.g., highlighting marketing, market share, cost control, and efficiency issues) (Coddington, Palmquist & Trollinger, 1985; Rosenstein, 1986).

Hospitals also are finding new ways to obtain services (e.g., housekeeping) such as contracting-out, shared services, corporate parent provided services, among others. Sometimes these approaches tie into changes in the organizational structure, as when a function is "lopped off" and relocated outside the organization. Furthermore, strategic decisions can result in changes in the designation of personnel such that employees of the hospital, by the stroke of a pen, become employees of other entities. Similarly, advances in technology in combination with deliberate strategy can lead to changes in the definition of which diagnoses require hospitalization and which can be treated on an outpatient basis.

Hospitals, of course, are concerned about their revenue position and are adopting strategies to increase hospital market share. These include affiliation with health maintenance organizations and preferred provider organizations (PPOs). Other efforts focus on reducing the average length of stay through hospital-based programs that extend into the community, such as use of convalescent units and nursing homes. Another example is the use of wellness clinics to identify developing health conditions at an earlier stage in order to stem their progress and thus avoid long-term hospital stays. This is particularly advantageous in the era of the PPS, since hospitals stand to make the most money on patients who can be discharged relatively quickly.

Change probably also will occur in the decision-making process about hospital operations and development, the actors involved in these decisions, and the criteria used (e.g., with regard to the adoption of new technology or determining staffing levels). Identifying where and why change will occur is greatly complicated by the fact that changes made within one area of a hospital may affect other areas, and that such impacts cannot always be foreseen.

TRENDS IN HOSPITAL TECHNOLOGY

The diffusion of new medical technology has occurred rapidly, with an increasing percentage of hospitals adopting the most sophisticated equipment. Intensive care units, which have become more numerous, are just one instance of such diffusion. Technological change within the hospital has been a major issue, frequently dealt with by a number of disciplines including management, economics, and sociology (Russell, 1979; Goldfarb et al., 1980; Gordon, MacEachron & Fisher, 1975; see Maxwell & Sapolsky, Chap. 11 of this book, and Kimberly et al., Chap. 12 of this book).

The impact of technology on staffing patterns depends on the characteristics of the technology. We need to differentiate analytically between the various levels and types of technology and the points at which hospitals adopted or expanded their use of specific technologies (Bernstein et al., 1975; Neuhauser, 1983). Dimensions to be considered include whether the item is a new adoption (an innovation) versus an expanded or curtailed use of an established technology; related to prevention, diagnosis, therapy, or rehabilitation; a major or minor investment; complex or simple; widespread or limited in application; or labor intensive or labor reducing. Time is another important dimension since technological impacts can occur immediately or on a lagged basis.

The introduction of leading-edge technology may have very different implications for the institution compared to those resulting from the continued use of an established technology. For example, when a new technology is brought on-line, the hospital may not be able to shift or reduce staff involved in the use of established technology because the new technology may not reduce, let alone eliminate, the need for existing technology. This is potentially the case for a range of halfway technologies, for example, dialysis or, in an earlier time, the iron lung, that maintain but cannot restore capacity for the patient (Thomas, 1971, 1974; Maxwell, 1986). Also, the adoption of new technology may increase rather than decrease the need for additional hospital services (a multiplier effect). The result is that the adoption of new technology may produce a need for additional staff and therefore increase the staff-to-patient ratio.

The definition of what constitutes appropriate levels of use for a variety of well-established technologies has changed over the past few decades. Definitional changes relate both to the proportion of patients treated with a given technology as well as to the number of procedures per patient for a given technology. Increasing the number of procedures per patient probably leads to increases in staff-to-patient ratios. However, the reverse situation—declining utilization of a specific technology—may not result in a reduction in staff-to-patient ratios.

Compared to such factors as administrative requirements, regulation, and care intensity, technological developments probably have accounted for the largest share of growth in staff-to-patient ratios over time. Differences in the use and adoption of technology probably also explain most of the differences noted in the rate of growth in this ratio among different types of hospitals.

The presence of intensive care units should be considered separately from technology *per se* as a factor in the growth of staff-to-patient ratios over time. While there clearly is an overlap because of the range and complexity of the technology involved in intensive care, there are distinct differences. The introduction, expansion, or reduction of special units providing more intensive care can alter staffing requirements even if some of the technology associated with such care does not represent a change from that already in place in the hospital.

Factors related to this source of change in staff-to-patient ratios include the type of unit, when it was introduced, the type of technology in use, the labor intensity of that technology (i.e., associated staff-to-patient ratios), and the number of beds. Of course, the technology involved in intensive care may also change, and there are thus two distinct causes associated with changes in ICU staffing patterns.

TRENDS IN HOSPITAL COSTS

Labor traditionally has been the single largest hospital expense, accounting for more than half of all costs. However, there are variations by hospital type. Thus, in 1986 the proportion of expenditures for labor was 54% for all nonfederal short-term hospitals combined. It was approximately the same for two of the subcategories, not-for-profit and state and local government hospitals. However, in the third subcategory, for-profit hospitals, nonlabor costs exceeded labor costs starting in 1975, and by 1986 labor accounted for only 43% of total costs. It is interesting that the percentage of total costs devoted to labor was by far the lowest in for-profit hospitals. This is a striking contrast to the case presented by other types of hospitals. As just noted, labor was 54% of all costs in the overall short-term category. It accounted for 56% of total costs for all U.S. hospitals combined, and 65–75% in the various categories of long-term and federal hospitals (American Hospital Association, 1987, Table 1).

The relatively low percentage of total costs devoted to labor in for-profit hospitals may reflect a less-expensive mix of personnel combined with lower staff-to-patient ratios compared to those of other types of nonfederal short-term hospitals. In sharp contrast, long-term and federal hospitals expend far higher percentages of their total costs for labor as compared to other types of hospitals, because of the labor-intensive nature of their operations.

One analysis of hospital costs attributes their rise from 1955 to 1975 to increases in nonlabor costs per patient day, earnings per employee, and the number of employees per patient day (Feldstein, 1981). Interestingly, it was the nonlabor factors that contributed most to the overall rise in hospital costs. Growth in nonlabor costs resulted primarily from increases in the volume rather than the price of nonlabor inputs. By contrast, the largest share of labor cost growth resulted from increases in earnings per employee.

Labor costs declined steadily from 1960 to 1975 as a percentage of total hospital costs per patient day. Feldstein's data, which are based on a subset of hospitals and use payroll alone as the measure of labor costs, show that labor had fallen from 62% to 53% of total costs by 1975. If total labor costs (employee benefits plus payroll) are examined for all U.S. hospitals, then, from 1971 to 1986 the cost of labor dropped from 67% to 56% of the average cost per patient day (American Hospital Association, 1987, Table 1). From 1972 to 1986, benefits rose from 8% to 15% of total hospital labor costs, making the inclusion of this item essential. Clearly, however, labor costs have dropped as a percentage of total hospital expenditures while the role of nonlabor inputs has increased (Gold-farb et al., 1980; Feldstein, 1981).

POLICY ISSUES AND SUGGESTED TOPICS FOR RESEARCH

The concept of organizational functioning relative to the external environment and to changes that occur in that environment leads to questions about how hospitals will alter their behavior to adjust to their changing environment. A primary question is how hospitals, as organizations functioning in the expansion-prone environment that existed until recently, gave rise to the observed staffing patterns. Furthermore, what impact will the greater scarcity of resources and cost-consciousness have on future trends in the number of hospital personnel, in staffing ratios, and on hospital performance? We do not yet have available the necessary data to identify with certainty what kinds of staffing adjustments are imminent and how they will affect the quality of care.

What are the implications of the continuing growth in staff-to-patient ratios for organizational decisions about future staffing? Will hospitals introduce cost-benefit analysis as a standard tool in making staffing and technology decisions? Will there be a moderation or reversal of the historically visible pattern of continuing increases in staff-to-patient ratios? Important policy issues relate to the answers to these questions.

Since the 1970s, concern for the increasing cost of inpatient care has focused heavily on technological changes in health care delivery and their implications (Goldfarb et al., 1980). However, the historical data reviewed indicate that, despite the changes in the relative contribution of labor and technology to total cost, staff-to-patient ratios increased even during the years of heightened concern with technological development. A significant proportion of the ratio increase probably can be attributed to the implementation of new technology. The increased availability of intensive care and administrative and regulatory requirements such as those related to Medicare also undoubtedly were major factors. Apparently, however, advances in medical technology are making medical care more, rather than less, labor intensive. Consequently, the introduction of new technology into the institutional medical setting must be analyzed in terms of its impact on staffing requirements, including effects on staffing levels and ratios as well as on occupational mix.

In addition to the other cost impacts of technology, it can be assumed that related increases in the intensity of hospital labor have been a factor in increasing costs per patient day. The question therefore can be raised: If technological improvements increase rather than decrease the unit cost of producing inpatient services, where do the added benefits of the care improvements appear relative to their cost? Presumably, this relates to professional assumptions about the value of providing better care. If this is the answer, it focuses concern on the difference between hospitals and other economic entities in the criteria used for adding technology and staff.

The general model used by manufacturing organizations to justify the adoption of new process technology or the hiring of additional staff reflects an expectation that such changes will produce benefits that exceed the costs to the organization. In this regard, the ability to define and quantify the value of the end product as well as the cost of its manufacture makes it possible both to assess unit costs and to measure product improvements.

Difficulty in defining the end product is among the problems faced by medical care in general and hospital care in particular (Shapleigh, 1985; see Riley & Brehm, Chap. 4 of this book). That, in combination with the retrospective reimbursement policy that prevailed until Medicare shifted to a Prospective Payment System (PPS), resulted in an industry approach that favored accepting any improvement in the ability to diagnose or treat patients as a benefit worth the cost. This appears to have affected not only technological but also staffing decisions. For example, the justification for additional nursing staff was based on a model of nursing functions, not on an assessment of its impact on staff-to-patient ratios, and, as a result, on the unit cost of care. If, consequently, the cost of care rose, this was passed along in additional billing. If the mix of patients treated required more care, thus raising the staff-to-patient ratio, the increased cost also could be passed along to insurers. Medicare's shift to the PPS and the increasingly competitive nature of the market have forced the hospital industry to become more concerned about the cost of caring for a patient and the factors that may affect this cost. This raises important policy issues concerning the adoption of new technology and the addition of staff.

A major issue in regard to the long-term growth in staff-to-patient ratios and its potential impact on efforts to control hospital inpatient care costs is the relationship between these ratio increases and changes in the amount and quality of care provided. If, as suggested, a major part of these ratio increases was related to the adoption of new technology (Aries & Kennedy, 1986), then we must consider the potential impact on both technology and staffing of the PPS, a reimbursement approach that may become the standard in the industry. How will a potentially modified orientation toward the assessment of costs versus benefits, including increases in the quality of care, which is driven by a change in reimbursement approach, affect new adoptions or expanded use of technology and the interplay of staff and technology? Will future technology decisions reflect concerns for the effect on the staff-to-patient ratio?

The impact of prospective payment on future staff-to-patient ratios will depend partly on the standard used when reimbursement levels are changed under the system. This should affect hospitals' responses both to prospective reimbursement and to changes in the inpatient care market. In the long run, the standard for determining DRG payment levels will have to be some measure of hospital performance. Basing it on a general average will have implications different from basing it on ''industry leaders,'' the most price- and cost-competitive hospitals, or some derived model. The relationship between how reimbursement levels are set for the PPS and the staff-to-patient ratios has implications for the cost as well as the quality of care.

Along with the observed growth in staffing ratios, labor categories have been redefined in terms of duties and job titles (see Riley & Brehm, Chap. 4 of this book). It is important to consider what these changes suggest about future trends in hospital staffing. Possibilities, as discussed, include the use of more highly trained and skilled staff as well as the deskilling of some work.

The growth in the staff-to-patient ratio occurred, for the most part, against a backdrop of hospital concern for improving the quality of care that was largely unrestrained by any external requirements for cost/benefit analyses. The recent reductions in hospital patient days and, from 1983 to 1985, in staff size, also undoubtedly affected staff-to-patient ratios. Recently, however, we have entered a new era in which cost, utilization control, and market competition can be expected to play a much greater role in shaping care, staffing, and technology decisions.

Any future cuts in either staff or staffing ratios will occur within the context reflecting both current conditions and the history of long-term increases in these factors. Staffing cuts may have important implications for the ability to provide appropriate care, for the adoption and use of new technology, and for effective managerial and administrative approaches within different types of hospitals. Important questions arise. How will the hospitals that developed under the old conditions respond to the new, cost conscious, competitive environment? Will efforts for cost and utilization control result in efficient staff cuts based on market forces? Will it be necessary to monitor or regulate staff cuts to assure that they do not unduly restrict the delivery of appropriate care and the introduction of valuable new technology?

NOTES

1. The data through 1986 do not reflect a change in this persistent pattern because of the impact of the Prospective Payment System (PPS) under Medicare and the general movements for reduction of inpatient care, competition in the health care market, and cost control in medical care. Data in Table 1, *Hospital Statistics* (American Hospital Association, 1987) show FTE personnel/100 adjusted average daily census. It is possible to compute the FTE staff-to-patient ratio for certain hospital categories from data in Table 1 using the unadjusted figures. Ratios based on adjusted figures appear systematically lower. However, adjusted data are not available for the "Total United States" category nor before 1970–72 for some hospital categories.

2. This figure is substantially lower than might have been the case because of the effect of nonfederal psychiatric hospitals, which in 1965 made a high relative contribution to average daily census but had a very low FTE-per-100 patients figure. Deinstitutionalization reduced the average daily census over the years, but the FTE per 100 patients increased almost fivefold in less than 20 years.

3. Nonfederal short-term general and other special hospitals is a category almost

identical to "community hospitals." It adds to "community hospitals" the small number of "hospital units of institutions" of which there were 50 in 1986. The disadvantage of using the "community hospital" category itself is that this data series did not start until 1972.

10

Health Care Technology Market Testing and Marketing: An Industry Perspective

John L. Fanton and Ronna Borenstein-Levy

This chapter offers the reader an industry perspective on health care technology market testing and marketing. Medical technology in the 20th century has made possible remarkable advances in health care—diagnostic breakthroughs, exponential increases in basic medical knowledge, and therapeutic wonders. Until very recently, such benefits were more than enough to justify whatever the costs were to develop, purchase, and maintain this technology. Today this is no longer true.

The cost of health care is now uppermost in the minds of government policymakers, insurance executives, health care administrators, and medical manufacturers. Along with all other aspects of the health care delivery system, medical instrumentation must now be justified not only by what it does for the patient but also what it does to the budget. This is not surprising, considering the fact that the United States currently spends $425 billion on health care each year (*Newsweek*, January 26, 1987).

This chapter will focus on one company, Hewlett-Packard (HP), which markets over 350 major medical products and systems. Its purpose is to elucidate some of the concerns and priorities that now govern HP's activities in the development, manufacturing, and marketing of these products. One of our major objectives is to demonstrate that, in order to be successful in today's environment, manufacturers of medical products cannot conduct their business operations in a vacuum. The success of the effort relies on a dependable process of feedback and cooperation from the health care providers themselves.

In order to appreciate how important this process is, let us first look at the power of medical technology and imagine the consequences if it were allowed to develop without this feedback and evaluation. Modern medical technology has made a significant impact on the epidemiology and definition of disability, morbidity, and mortality. But in other respects as well, the impact of its proliferation has been staggering. The expectations of patients or consumers have become more demanding; the job descriptions of the nurse, the doctor, and other health care practitioners have been altered; medical school curricula have been rewritten; and government and regulatory roles have been redefined. One cannot underestimate the impact of technology's proliferation.

Then there are the ethical considerations. How much technology is enough, and how much is too much? When should we intervene, and when should we withhold intervention? Who should pay the bill, and what happens if there is no one to pay it? One of these questions in particular points to a fundamental controversy concerning the proliferation of modern medical technology. Dr. Michael DeBakey expressed it very directly. In response to the question "How much technology is enough?" he said:

I don't really know how much is enough technology; I can tell you this, when we're dealing with patients and when we're dealing with a patient's family, their response to this would be "as much as is necessary to get our loved one restored to normal life." And that's about the only answer I can give. (DeBakey, 1976)

While not all of us would agree with this opinion, we would all share Dr. DeBakey's sensitivity to the ethics of the question. That is why it is so important that manufacturers of medical technology manage their activities not only within the context of business responsibility but also within the framework of social responsibility.

With this introduction, let us turn now to the specific challenges medicine and medical equipment manufacturers face. First, remember that the mandates imposed by government regulation, cost-containment directives, and other guidelines for the practice of medicine are not new. Rather, they are as old as the medical profession itself—one early example being the Hippocratic oath. It serves no purpose to list the many laws and regulations that have been passed concerning regulation of medicine. Let it suffice to say that it is an area that has long been subject to government and legislative intervention.

In the present DRG environment, what alternatives are there for the health care provider and the medical manufacturer? The question becomes how best to research, develop, and utilize technology that will truly contribute to higher quality and economic efficiencies of health care, and at the same time eliminate technology that imposes costs not commensurate with derived benefit.

To save costs, the health care provider could decide not to use life-saving technology, and thereby reduce the quality of care. Or the provider could decide not to use this technology for everyone, and thereby reduce availability of services. Most will agree that, at least in contemporary U.S. society, these are not viable alternatives.

Is it not preferable for the health care provider to offer high-quality health care while at the same time improving the efficiency with which this health care is provided and thereby controlling costs? Most providers have already adopted this objective in an effort to offer quality services and remain competitive in a dynamic health care environment.

As a result, health care providers have made significant changes in the type of services offered and even in the locations where they are offered. And the requirements for medical technology now exceed the basic need for sophisticated measurements and analysis.

Modern medicine requires equipment that offers quality, accuracy, and reliability as well as gives the hospital a competitive advantage and improves the staff's efficiency while keeping the cost of ownership low. Medical clinicians need equipment that will help them to make faster and better decisions and to share information among departments and offices inside and outside the hospital. Moreover, there is a need for a responsive service and support organization to minimize equipment downtime. HP was able to define these marketplace priorities through a formal program of market research and testing and as a result of the relationships that we have built over the years with our customers. And HP is now addressing these issues in its product marketing plans.

HP is just one example of a major medical manufacturer that has established a strong marketing program driven by the marketplace. We use HP examples because these are the ones we know best. HP does not enter into any technology without a significant amount of research.

Let us begin with market testing and research. At this point the following questions must be answered: what does the medical provider need? who will use the equipment? where will it be used? and most importantly, will the technology really work the way it is intended?

HP's marketing personnel work closely with research and development engineers to ensure that the answers to these questions are found. Formal textbook research is conducted. The marketplace and potential customers are surveyed. HP's sales force is consulted, and focus groups are held. The purpose of a focus group is to identify the concerns of a particular market segment by interviewing a small group of people who are characteristic of the target marketplace as a whole. While not a statistical sample, such groups provide insight into the opinions, needs, and wants of potential customers.

Many other research projects are also undertaken. For example, HP organizes internship programs whereby our employees work side by side with physicians and nurses to learn how the technology is used.

We ask nurses and doctors to serve as consultants. And HP has a dedicated government affairs manager whose job is to ensure that technology responds to all government and legislative requirements and that HP remains aware of proposed legislative and regulatory changes. Finally, clinical test sites are selected where equipment is tested by hospitals in real-life settings so that marketing and engineering can obtain feedback on its performance.

In general, HP's research has allowed the company to define the overall essential qualities of medical instrumentation for today's health care environment. Those essential qualities are the following:

First and foremost, a technological contribution should make possible a true clinical advancement. An HP example is the quality of the cardiac ultrasound images. The continued improvement in image quality has allowed physicians to diagnose more rapidly and accurately cardiac abnormalities. Pathology that might have been difficult or impossible to visualize is now clearly visible.

Second, equipment should save time and labor. Labor, by some estimates, accounts for over 60% of a hospital's budget. Equipment that speeds service delivery, enables one staff person to handle more patients at a time, and cuts down on the demands of recordkeeping is going to save money. An HP example is the Obstetrical Management System that makes it possible for nurses to provide monitoring and surveillance for several ambulatory obstetrical patients at the same time, all accomplished from a central station.

A third essential quality of medical instrumentation is reliability. Using defibrillators as an example, reliability not only saves time and money but also saves lives. Greater reliability and accuracy can also mean faster tests, fewer repeated tests, more precise diagnoses, and the avoidance of unnecessary further tests, hospital days, and procedures. Reliability also means less money spent on supplies and maintenance and less staff time devoted to babysitting undependable equipment.

A fourth quality is functional versatility. This is demonstrated by the many new medical systems that now include a personal computer as an integral part of the product. The availability of industry-standard personal computers means that when the equipment is not being used for medical applications it can be used to run a variety of office automation software programs that can improve nursing and administrative productivity.

Fifth, compatibility and upgradability of equipment is also essential to assure that as new technological advances come along, the hospital does not have to scrap all of its earlier models. One example of this strategy for HP is the Ultrasound Imaging product line. HP designed its imaging systems to keep pace with state-of-the-art developments. The flexible electronic architecture allows new technological developments to be integrated into the existing piece of equipment so that the customer doesn't have to buy a new system in order to obtain the newest capabilities. Every HP phased-array ultrasound imaging system ever produced can be upgraded to the features and capabilities of the most sophisticated systems sold today for a fraction of the cost of a new system.

And finally, ease of use is a very important quality. User-friendly design features are an important contributor to productivity in the hospital and help to minimize training and retraining costs.

Thus, the first strategic step for the medical manufacturer is to conduct research to determine marketplace needs. The second step is to respond to those needs in product design. Finally, a plan is designed to position the company and its products in the marketplace. It is this market positioning that will be reviewed now.

Based on marketplace research, HP believes that advanced technology is no longer a strong market stimulus by itself. Customers have indicated, through conversation and through formal research, that advanced technology is just the beginning. And therefore, that idea constitutes the framework of HP's medical marketing positioning program: *advanced technology is just the beginning.*

Promotional literature and HP's sales force now communicate more than technology. The issues of quality, reliability, efficiency, low cost of ownership, and comprehensive training, service, and support are all important elements in HP's agenda.

For example, let us isolate one of these positioning strategies—low cost of ownership. This is a very important concept in today's environment.

Total cost of ownership encompasses much more than the initial purchase price of the equipment, which is only the tip of the iceberg. True cost of ownership includes the cost of consumable accessories and supplies, maintenance, training and retraining staff, the actual life span of the product, the costs incurred from downtime or inaccuracy, the motivation of staff to use it, and ultimately, its impact on patient care.

The design criteria that were discussed as being essential qualities of medical instrumentation will melt this iceberg to a size that can be managed by today's and tomorrow's resources. HP's fetal monitor technology is one example of how the company has addressed this cost-of-ownership issue.

HP fetal monitors have contributed to many advancements in obstetrical care. First introduced by HP in 1967, this equipment has continued to evolve and improve over the years. When it was introduced, the product was very complicated to use and maintain. Today, HP's recent fourth-generation fetal monitor not only incorporates the latest technology but is also easy to set up and use.

Fetal heart rate can be found much faster, more reliably, and can be continuously monitored for hours with little staff attention. What makes all this productive innovation possible are three HP microprocessors. The large digital processing capability makes the monitor not only faster and more reliable but also means fewer circuits, lower power requirements, and lower operating temperature—all leading to overall improvements in reliability.

In one improved medical instrument we have seen labor and time saving, increased accuracy and reliability, ease of use, and greatly reduced maintenance costs—all of which improve the hospital's bottom line.

Another marketing tool, born out of our customer focus groups, is HP's comprehensive support services: training, consultation, installation, and servicing. Installation specialists work with the hospital to prepare a convenient, personalized installation plan. HP's product-training programs are professionally designed to develop confidence in each equipment user so that productivity does not lose momentum during installation.

A flexible service and support program also includes a North American Telephone Response Center, which can connect with the hospital's medical computer system for remote troubleshooting. If the problem cannot be solved over the phone, a support engineer is then dispatched to the facility.

HP also offers continuing-education credits for application seminars in topics like pressure measurement and fetal monitoring. Finally, HP features a biomedical partnership program that trains and supports hospital biomedical engineers to perform adjustments and repairs. This integration of hospital and HP resources for system support lowers the cost of ownership while maintaining a high degree of protection and customer satisfaction. In many sales situations it is the added value of HP's comprehensive support programs that differentiates the company from its competition.

Another marketing imperative that has become increasingly important in this age of DRGs deserves a brief note. This is the requirement for extensive documentation that must be provided to hospital decision makers before they can purchase equipment. Because cost is a key issue, HP provides data on the long-term cost of ownership of the product, upgrade opportunities and costs, service contracts and their costs, and even researches the reimbursement issues associated with a new technology. This data is provided in addition to the usual product feature and benefit information. Of course, detailed service manuals, application notes, and extensive training material are provided as well.

However, the most important feature of HP's marketing program is our ongoing customer relationships. HP identifies the key decision makers in health care today as the physician, nurse manager, hospital administrator, biomedical engineer, and purchasing agent. Each of these people has different priorities and different needs. And HP must respond to each in his or her own language.

We use participation in major medical conventions and trade shows, such as those of the American Heart Association, American College of Cardiology, and American Association of Critical Care Nurses, as an opportunity to talk with these customers. Whenever possible, company representatives participate as speakers in programs that these professional organizations sponsor and in programs offered by universities for the purpose of creating an information exchange. HP also provides support for the continuing-education programs that are run by many of the professional medical associations. Finally, HP executives frequently visit customer sites to understand first-hand the changes in health care.

It is HP's belief that medical manufacturers should be active partners in the health care business. They must keep their eye on the marketplace in order to fulfill their business and social responsibility: to introduce only those products that are truly needed, and at the same time not hold back the progress of technology merely to reduce costs. It is a delicate balance.

The final phase of a medical manufacturer's marketing plan should be based on feedback and evaluation. Customers' verbal feedback gives an indication of how well a manufacturer is doing relative to business and social responsibilities. But another kind of feedback, buying behavior, is just as strong an indication. It would be naive to try to hide the fact that profit is a critical measure of any marketing plan. In fact, HP considers the profit objective to be so important that it is listed first among the goals in our corporate framework for success. HP believes that, without profit, a company is unable to meet any of its other obligations to employees, to customers, or to society as a whole.

The purchasing behavior of the marketplace, together with its verbal feedback, provides the public consent needed to carry on with the corporate mission as a medical manufacturer.

In conclusion, the future of medical technology depends on a cooperative effort of both the users and the providers of this equipment. Each must do his or her job with an ultimate goal in mind: the life of the patient. Industry and clinicians must work together to ensure that the most modern technology is made available to all who could benefit from it, balancing the associated costs with the potential therapeutic results. And both must cooperate in an aggressive effort to develop creative solutions that respond to the growing cost of delivering these services. To quote from columnist Jake Page, writing in *Science* (1982): "To moan about new technologies disrupting the social order—instead of thinking about how to make new technologies work better—is to look at your hand and wish it were a paw." Medical technology cannot and should not go back, but must move forward in a socially responsible and united effort.

11

Prospective Payment in the ESRD Program: Implications for Technology and Program Administration

James H. Maxwell and Harvey M. Sapolsky

In October 1983, the Medicare program changed its method for reimbursing the hospital services provided to its beneficiaries. Since its inception in 1966, Medicare had paid hospitals on a retrospective basis. That is, it reimbursed hospitals for all reasonable costs incurred in providing care to Medicare patients. Under the new system, known as the Prospective Payment System (PPS), Medicare sets the price for 467 diagnoses and pays hospitals only those amounts irrespective of the costs that are incurred in providing care. The intent of the prospective system is to encourage hospitals to become efficient and thus control Medicare expenditures.

The federal government was not altogether without experience with prospective payment. The end-stage renal disease (ESRD) program, a Social Security administered benefit for victims of kidney failure, has used a preestablished price for dialysis services since its inception in 1973. In Section 2991 of the 1972 Social Security amendments, Congress mandated that the federal government finance the treatment of chronic renal disease. Because the great expense involved had prevented many victims from being treated, the law made the federal government a monopsonist buyer for a service not then being widely offered. The ESRD program's use of a uniform flat charge for each dialysis session represented the first time that Medicare had paid something other than all reasonable costs incurred for authorized services (Lowrie & Hampers, 1984). Medicare officials hoped that the fixed fee would provide incentives for facilities to control their expenses and thus the expenditures of the ESRD program (Rettig & Marks, 1980).

This chapter examines the origins and lessons of the ESRD payment methodology. During the ESRD program's history, Medicare officials increasingly experimented with prospective payment as a method of reimbursing both facilities and physicians. Early supporters believed the program might serve as a precedent for national health insurance. Instead, as the first federal health program to utilize prospective payment methods, the ESRD program offers insights about the advantages and disadvantages of incentive reimbursement mechanisms, especially those implemented by the government. It thus serves as a prototype for Medicare's current cost-control efforts and possibly for the future implementation of a reimbursement system in which other payers of health care services participate.

ORIGINS OF ESRD PAYMENT ARRANGEMENTS

The ESRD program provides a near-universal entitlement to treatment for individuals of all ages suffering from chronic renal failure. The vast majority of patients receive hemodialysis treatment, a procedure that removes excess waste products and fluid from a patient's blood by circulating it through an artificial kidney called a dialyzer. Hemodialysis is performed either on an inpatient basis, at dedicated outpatient facilities, or at home. Peritoneal dialysis, a much less utilized method, involves the use of the patient's own peritoneum membrane rather than an artificial kidney to eliminate solutes and fluid from the circulation. The third major treatment for kidney failure is transplantation, which requires the surgical removal of a kidney from either a living relative or a cadaver and its placement in a patient.

Officials at the Department of Health, Education, and Welfare (HEW) confronted a formidable challenge in implementing a payment program for kidney disease. The department had only seven months from the passage of the kidney disease amendment to devise a payment policy for all the medical services provided to patients (Blagg, 1977). Facilities had to be convinced that adequate reimbursement was forthcoming; otherwise they would not provide the life-saving treatment (Kusserow, 1982). The problem was compounded by the fact that many of the facilities that provided long-term maintenance dialysis in the early 1970s were not financially stable. The overriding goal of the reimbursement policy was to offer facilities financial incentives not only to continue but to expand their services to meet the anticipated increase in demand. Cost control and quality assurance, though important, were secondary objectives of the payment policy (Rettig, 1980).

The federal government's lack of experience as the sole payer for a life-saving treatment created administrative obstacles to the design of payment policy. Management responsibility for the financing of care resided with the Bureau of Health Insurance (BHI) of the Social Security Administration (Rettig, 1982). Because the Public Health Service had been the lead federal agency for monitoring renal treatments prior to 1972, the BHI had little familiarity with issues related to kidney disease. Also, neither the kidney amendments nor their legislative history provided detailed guidance for the program in charting a reimbursement policy (U.S. Congress, Senate, 1972).[1]

From the start, officials recognized that the new program required a departure from Medicare's traditional cost-based payment methodology. It was already obvious by the early 1970s that retrospective reimbursement was in large part responsible for Medicare's soaring expenditures (Feldstein, 1966).[2] Congress had considered a change to prospective payment for the entire Medicare program in its deliberations over the 1972 Social Security amendments, and actually took preliminary steps toward such a system by establishing limits on per-diem hospital costs and authorizing experiments with prospective payment (U.S. Congress, Senate, 1972). Yet, opposition from hospitals and Medicare's lack of administrative experience with alternative-payment policies prevented their adoption in 1972.[3] The ESRD program thus offered a unique opportunity for reimbursement reform, which was not available to the larger program.

Without some form of control on payment, government officials feared the costs of the dialysis program would be several times the estimates presented to the Congress when the legislation was being considered.[4] They believed that the kidney disease amendment required a total review of coverage policies for transplantation and dialysis due to the expense of these therapies and the certain disappearance of a non-Medicare population as a base of comparison for Medicare's charges. The disappearance of a private patient population was especially important as BHI officials had been relying on comparisons to determine the level of reasonable charges in paying for health care services provided to federal beneficiaries (Rettig & Marks, 1980). The staff had considerable latitude in designing a payment methodology because the 1972 amendments had given the HEW secretary discretionary authority for implementing the program.

Although there was agreement on the need to limit costs, there was initially no consensus on how this was to be accomplished. BHI officials considered several alternative-payment methods for outpatient facilities, including fixed fees per treatment session, limits on the costs per hour of treatment, and a competitive contracting process in which the government would purchase services from the lowest bidder in a service region (Rettig & Marks, 1980). The BHI decided to reimburse for dialysis on a per-treatment basis up to an established "screen" or limit. By not selecting competitive contracting, the government relinquished some of its potential monopsony power and almost certainly paid a higher price for dialysis services than would have been possible with contracting (Bovbjerg, Held & Pauley, 1982). The screen may, however, have been the most feasible payment method, causing the least disruption in Medicare's traditional administrative and reimbursement practices.

It proved even more difficult to determine a level for a screen than to choose a payment methodology. Cost data on dialysis services were not readily available (Blagg, 1977; Rettig, 1980).[5] Data varied widely with facility charges ranging from $11,000 to $48,000 per patient per year. A medical task force organized by the National Kidney Foundation suggested that dialysis charges should be limited to a range of $120 to $150 per treatment (Rettig & Marks, 1980). The lack of legislative authority to reimburse facilities for their capital costs presented policymakers with yet another dilemma. To ensure an adequate supply of dialysis facilities, the Bureau of Health Insurance had to set the per-treatment screen at a level that would cover not only the operating costs of providing dialysis treatment but also the costs of constructing and starting up a facility. As one official put it, they decided to set the screen at the level that would be incurred by an economical provider operating under prevailing market conditions.[6]

The draft regulations issued in June 1973 suggested that limits on per-treatment costs were likely, but did not contain a specific numerical value (U.S. Congress, Senate, 1982b). Following the publication of the draft, officials prepared a letter to fiscal intermediaries that included instructions for implementing an "interim" program as well as a screen on allowable facility charges. In the interim program, Medicare agreed to pay 80% of the average costs of outpatient treatment at either a hospital-based or a freestanding facility, up to a screen of $150 per treatment (U.S. Congress, Senate, 1982a). (Many state Medicaid programs began paying the remaining 20% of the facility charge for those patients who met their eligibility requirements.) Though the screen was originally intended as an upper limit on per-treatment costs, it soon became the standard fee for most facilities. In contrast, Medicare reimbursed for home dialysis on a reasonable cost basis, relying to the extent possible on its standard payment procedures (U.S. Congress, Senate, 1982a).

The BHI's commitment to cost control was not, however, absolute. The agency announced that exceptions to the screen on outpatient charges were possible if a facility could either demonstrate hardship or that its costs exceeded the $150 limit. In practice, Medicare's intermediaries routinely granted hospitals exemptions to the cost screen without evidence of justifiably higher costs (Prottas & Sapolsky, 1980; Prottas & Sapolsky, 1981). The exception system was administered loosely to enlist the cooperation of hospitals and to ensure that enough facilities provided treatment. The exception system thus became the major loophole in the fixed-payment system (Prottas & Sapolsky, 1980; Prottas & Sapolsky, 1981). Indeed, by the late 1970s, the majority of hospitals were being reimbursed on the basis of reasonable costs (Eggers, 1984).[7]

Another question confronting the program was how to pay for physician services. This turned out to be a more politically sensitive issue than facility reimbursement. Because maintenance dialysis was not provided directly by physicians, there was great uncertainty about what to pay doctors for their routine supervision of care (Rettig & Marks, 1980). No satisfactory precedent existed because third-party insurers had been paying physicians widely varying amounts (Blagg, 1977; Lowrie & Hampers, 1981). Medicare officials believed that fee for service was unwarranted given the fact that physicians had only a supervisory role in dialysis care. They favored a capitation approach that would limit the total amount of physician reimbursement. Yet at the start of the program, the capitation approach was politically unacceptable to physician groups, most especially to the American Medical Association. Medicare officials then proposed that physicians receive payment directly from the facility in which they supervise care, as part of overhead, with the actual fee set by the facility (Rettig & Marks, 1980). Physicians viewed this arrangement as a threat to professional autonomy; they had no desire to bargain for salary with facilities providing treatment. Under intense political pressure from physician groups, the BHI devised an "alternative physician reimbursement method" that created a monthly capitation fee per patient, subject to the requirement that all doctors in a facility accept the same payment mechanism. In less than a year, physician groups accepted a capitation arrangement that had previously been an anathema—thus initiating the federal government's first experiment with prospective payment for physician services.

In contrast, the ESRD program relied on standard Medicare practices for reimbursing both inpatient dialysis and renal transplants (Bovbjerg, Held & Pauley, 1982). The use of a fixed fee per treatment was thought not feasible for patients sick enough to require hospitalization. It would have been difficult to establish a uniform price for patients with varying medical complications. In comparison to dialysis, transplantation involved a relatively small number of patients. With the financial implications of transplants limited by the number of available kidney donors, officials perceived less need for wholesale changes in payment policy. Reimbursements for transplants thus were based on a reasonable cost system, with Medicare paying 80% of the usual and customary charges (U.S. Congress, Senate, 1981). Services covered by the ESRD program included the costs of organ acquisition, tissue typing, organ preservation, and surgical transplantation. To encourage kidney donation, Medicare covered all operative and postoperative expenses for donors, without deductibles. BHI officials experimented with yet another payment methodology by using relative values to set surgeons' fees for renal transplants. In this methodology, Medicare paid physicians fees equal to those of surgeons performing other comparable procedures (U.S. Congress, Senate, 1982a).

PROGRAM GROWTH

Innovative reimbursement methods notwithstanding, the ESRD program has vastly exceeded the original cost estimates. Congress had been told that the program would require $100 million annual budgets, but by 1974, reimbursements totalled $229 million, and by 1983, they had risen to nearly $1.9 billion. Analysis shows that more than 70% of the reimbursement growth resulted from an expanding patient enrollment, with the numbers of enrollees increasing from 16,000 in 1974 to over 76,000 in 1983 (see Table 11.1).

Cost increases can be attributed largely to the accumulation of patients and an extension of the clinically eligible. Whereas prior to passage of the 1972 amendments, dialysis was basically rationed according to social and medical

Table 11.1

Medicare Enrollment, Per Capita Reimbursement, and Per Capita Reimbursement in Constant Dollars for Persons with End-Stage Renal Disease, 1974–1984

Year	Enrollment		Reimbursement per enrollee		Amount in 1974 dollars
	Number in thousands	Percent change	Amount[1]	% change	
1974	16.0	---	$14,300	---	$14,300
1975	22.7	41.9	15,900	11.2	14,193
1976	28.9	27.3	17,700	11.3	14,423
1977	34.8	20.4	18,400	4.0	13,682
1978	43.1	23.9	18,500	0.5	12,690
1979	50.8	17.9	19,900	7.6	12,495
1980	57.8	13.8	21,600	8.5	12,226
1981	64.1	10.9	23,000	6.5	11,754
1982	72.8	13.6	22,800	-0.9	10,439
1983	76.0	04.4	24,800	8.8	10,446
1984	89.4	17.7	20,200	-18.6	8,011

[1]The amount includes reimbursements for all individuals eligible for benefits under the ESRD program. It includes payment for dialysis, transplantation, inpatient care, and physician services. The reimbursement data is also influenced by variations in dialysis practices, patient mortality, and HCFA's data collection methodology.

Sources: Eggers, 1984; Unpublished data from the Health Care Financing Administration, 1985.

criteria, the program's implementation removed these barriers to access. With financial constraints eliminated, the population receiving dialysis became older and poorer than before the enactment of the program (Rubin, 1984; Eggers, Connerton & McMullan, 1984). Physicians also extended the patient selection criteria from those suffering from primary kidney disease to those with renal failure due to secondary diseases, such as congestive heart failure, hypertension, diabetes, and arteriosclerosis (Halper, 1986). The United States, in contrast to European countries, has neither patient eligibility requirements nor a fixed budget for the treatment of kidney disease (Prottas, 1983). The door to care was wide open.

Despite rampant inflation in the health care sector, the payment for facilities remained constant at $150 per treatment until 1983. (Payment was $138 per treatment when the physician fee was excluded). After adjusting for inflation, treatment costs in facilities complying with the screen decreased by more than 50% in the decade from 1973 to 1983. The screen on facility reimbursement must be viewed as the major cost-control device constraining the growth in total program expenditures. The use of the flat-rate method of reimbursement prevented per-patient costs from rising rapidly despite the fact that the cost of hospital and medical services increased significantly over the decade (Rettig, 1980; Lowrie & Hampers, 1984; Eggers, 1984). Data show that while average benefit payments rose from $14,300 per person in 1974 to $24,800 in 1983, when inflation adjusted, the per-patient expenditures declined dramatically. As Table 11.2 indicates, the per-patient payments for ESRD in current dollars rose more slowly than health care expenditures per capita or hospital expenses per inpatient day.

IMPACTS OF PROSPECTIVE PAYMENT

Changes in Dialyzer Design and Use

At least in theory, the government's use of a flat per-session reimbursement fee creates strong incentives for dialysis service providers to adopt cost-reducing innovations. Under the fixed-payment system, when a facility reduces expenses, it retains the difference between its costs and the allowable screen; if costs exceed the screen, the extra expenditures must be absorbed. Prospective payment eliminates the incentives in the retrospective reimbursement system to use technology in order to generate additional revenues. In turn, pressure from facilities providing treatment should lead manufacturers to reduce the per-session cost of their products. No longer do manufacturers receive financial rewards for quality improvements regardless of their effectiveness.

In fact, the use of a fixed fee per treatment has caused facilities to reduce the length of dialysis sessions. Shorter treatments permit reductions in staffing costs per patient and more intense use of capital equipment (Brentano & Funck, 1985). One way to achieve shorter dialysis times has been the adoption of larger-surface-

Table 11.2
Costs and Per Capita Expenditures for End-Stage Renal Disease Compared with Other Economic Indicators

| Year | Costs of the ESRD Program | | | | | Average Annual Payments | | | |
| | Amount in millions | Deflated to 1974 dollars | | ESRD benefits per enrollee | | Health care expenditures per capita | | Hospital expenses per inpatient day | |
		Composite Price Index	Medical Price Index	Amount	% change	Amount	% change	Amount	% change
1974	$228.5	$228	$228	$14,300	---	$522	---	$113	---
1975	361.1	330	322	15,900	11.2	591	14.8	133	17.6
1976	512.2	443	417	17,700	11.3	666	12.7	152	14.4
1977	641.3	521	477	18,400	4.0	743	11.6	173	13.8
1978	799.5	604	548	18,500	0.5	822	10.6	194	11.9
1979	1,009.7	685	634	19,900	7.6	920	11.9	216	11.3
1980	1,249.6	747	707	21,600	8.5	1,049	14.0	244	13.3
1981	1,471.1	797	752	23,000	6.5	1,197	14.1	284	16.4
1982	1,660.7	848	760	22,800	-0.9	1,334	11.4	327	15.1
1983	1,888.7	935	796	24,800	8.8	1,461	9.5	368	12.5
1984	1,805.4	857	716	20,200	-18.6	1,580	6.8	---	---

Sources: Eggers, 1984; U.S. Department of Health and Human Services, Health United States 1985; HCFA unpublished data, 1985.

area dialyzers and dialyzers with higher membrane permeability. The development of faster and more efficient dialyzers resulted from Scribner and his colleagues' clinical research, the so-called middle molecule hypothesis, which suggested that some features of uremia were caused by middle molecules in the range of 300–2,000 molecular weight (Hoenitch & Kerr, 1983). The clearance of these middle molecules required the development of dialyzers with either greater membrane surface area or membrane permeability (Chanard et al., 1985).

By adopting changes in technology that provided more-rapid clearance of solutes and higher ultrafiltration rates, facilities actually cut treatment times by more than half, from 10 to 12 hours in 1972 to 3 to 5 hours today (Brentano & Funck, 1985).[8] Assuming that nursing and technician expenses account for nearly 50% of per-treatment costs, one can then estimate that shorter dialysis times led to decreases in per-treatment costs on the order of 25%. Not only did shorter dialysis times generate savings for dialysis facilities, but they also led to greater patient comfort and convenience, allowing perhaps for fuller patient rehabilitation. Nonetheless, the absence of clinical guidelines for dialysis treatment times may have allowed certain facilities to reduce dialysis times without adopting more-efficient dialyzers (Drukker, 1983b).

Because dialyzers represent the single largest component of materials costs in the provision of dialysis, facilities have a major incentive to economize in their purchasing. One method of reducing purchases is for individuals to reuse their own dialyzers. (In order to be reused safely, a dialyzer must be carefully cleaned and sterilized, either manually or with an automated reprocessor, after each dialysis session.) (Deane & Bemis, 1983). Facilities that reuse dialyzers can realize savings estimated at between $2,000 and $6,000 per patient per year (Romeo, 1984). With such powerful financial incentives operating, the proportion of facilities reusing dialyzers has increased from 18% in 1976 to 58% in 1984.[9] Continued increases both in the proportion of facilities practicing reuse and in the average number of reuses performed can be expected.

The economic benefits of reuse must be weighed against the potential medical consequences. Patients often express concerns about medical effects, including infections and adverse immunologic reactions (Deane & Bemis, 1983; Romeo, 1984). They also fear that facilities may employ improper techniques in labeling and sterilizing dialyzers. However, the reuse of dialyzers has demonstrated its own therapeutic benefits, preventing "new dialyzer syndrome," a reaction to the first use of a dialyzer that causes respiratory distress, wheezing, back or chest pain, and chills or fever (Romeo, 1984). The exact magnitude and balance of benefits and risks resulting from reuse remains a subject of controversy.

Prospective payment systems create pressures on suppliers to be competitive in their pricing. In the case of dialysis services, a complex interaction has occurred between buyer pressure and reuse. By encouraging reuse and reducing overall sales of dialyzers, reimbursement policy led manufacturers to reduce their prices for dialyzers. According to Romeo, total sales for dialyzers declined by more than 40% from 1980 to 1983, largely as a result of reuse. In turn, Baxter

Travenol and other manufacturers decreased their prices for hollow-fiber dialyzers by as much as 56% in the same period.[10] Excess capacity in the supplier industry and improvements in manufacturing technology for hollow fibers made these price reductions possible.[11]

The U.S. reimbursement system clearly created an environment conducive to cost-saving innovation. The Japanese experience demonstrates what might have occurred with dialysis treatment had the ESRD program not adopted a fixed price per treatment. Japan initially used the U.S. system of per-treatment payments, and so faster, more efficient U.S.-made machines dominated their health care system (Vogel, 1979; Prottas & Sapolsky, 1980). The Japanese then instituted a system that paid for dialysis on a per-hour system explicitly to encourage providers to employ less-efficient Japanese products. The experience with renal transplantation provides a further indication of what might have occurred with dialysis treatment had the ESRD program not adopted a cost screen. Although the fee for dialysis services remained constant, per-patient reimbursements for renal transplants more than doubled as hospitals had no impetus to decrease expenses (Eggers, 1984).

Home Dialysis

Medicare officials initially considered home dialysis to be less expensive than center dialysis because it eliminated the need for nursing and technician care. During the program's establishment, some BHI officials even suggested mandating home dialysis whenever clinically feasible to save an estimated $10,000 per patient per year (Rettig & Marks, 1980). These officials were not its only supporters; many physicians, including the Seattle group that pioneered chronic maintenance dialysis, found that home dialysis offered patients a more normal life with greater opportunities for independence, rehabilitation, and employment (Blagg, 1977). Since the mid–1970s, policymakers have attempted to make reimbursement policy more conducive to home hemodialysis. Yet these efforts have so far proved ineffective in increasing the proportion of home dialysis patients.

Physician groups favoring home dialysis believed that the program's initial reimbursement policy inadvertently encouraged center dialysis (Blagg, 1977). At the start of the program neither facilities nor physicians received payment for patient training or the supervision of home care. Moreover, the home patient was not given coverage equivalent to those dialyzing in a facility. Patients dialyzing at home were faced with high out-of-pocket costs for equipment maintenance, necessary home modifications, utility bills, and the services of home aides. Self-dialyzing patients were also more likely to pay the 20% copayment for supplies than facility patients whose copayment obligations were often absorbed by the treatment center when not paid by Medicaid. The differences in the depth of coverage were the result of Medicare policy generally, which traditionally covered inpatient more generously than home care services, rather than attempts by BHI officials to discourage home dialysis (Rettig, 1982).

Based on the recommendations of physician groups, the BHI took a number of administrative actions to eliminate the reimbursement disincentives to home dialysis treatment. The agency expanded coverage for items used in home care, reimbursed for equipment installation and delivery, and instructed regional offices not to delay in providing payment to patients (Rettig & Marks, 1980). Fearful that financial considerations might encourage physicians to recommend in-center dialysis, BHI officials in April 1974 instituted a monthly retainer for physicians supervising home care. The fee was set at 70% of the payment for physicians supervising care in facilities, up to a maximum of $168 per patient per month. The retainer was supplemented by a flat fee for home dialysis training.

In addition, physician groups advocating home dialysis sought legislative changes in reimbursement policy. During the mid-1970s, several bills intended to increase home dialysis incentives were introduced and hearings were held, but Congress was reluctant to act (Rettig & Marks, 1980). While Congress deliberated the issues, the proportion of patients dialyzing at home decreased from more than 40% in 1972 to less than 16% in 1978 (Rubin, 1984).

Advocates of home dialysis believed that as many as 50% of patients could be safely treated in the home. The existence of wide geographic variations in the proportion of patients on home care, from a low of 2% in Rhode Island to more than 50% in Washington State, convinced them of the potential for home dialysis (Rettig, 1986). Those favoring home dialysis attributed these variations not to differences in patient characteristics or even to reimbursement policies directly but to differences in physician practice patterns and the type of facility ownership. Hospital facilities, for example, were twice as likely to initiate dialysis at home than freestanding facilities, which are typically part of large investor-owned chains (Davis, 1982).

In adopting the end-stage renal disease amendments of 1978, Congress sought to reverse the decline in the proportion of patients dialyzing at home and to reap the benefits of the wider use of this low-cost treatment setting. The amendment sponsors had initially proposed that 50% of all individuals suffering from kidney disease receive home dialysis (Rettig, 1982). However, political pressure from for-profit facilities had led to a weakening commitment to home dialysis in successive versions of the legislation (Rettig, 1982). Physicians operating for-profit dialysis facilities questioned the added burden placed on families of home patients and these patients' very chances of survival. They viewed government as interfering in the practice of medicine by promoting a medically inferior therapy (Lowrie & Hampers, 1984).

Although Congress did not adopt a national quota for home dialysis, it authorized modest changes in reimbursement policy. The legislation waived the three-month eligibility period for home and transplant patients. The law also provided 100% reimbursement for home hemodialysis equipment when managed by a facility. In place of a legislative quota for home care, Congress mandated "the maximum practical number of patients who are medically, socially, and psychologically suitable candidates for home dialysis or transplantation should be so treated" (Lowrie & Hampers, 1984).

The efforts to expand the number of patients on home hemodialysis through changes in payment policy were, however, overwhelmed by technical changes in dialysis therapy. In 1978, researchers at the University of Texas published a report on a new form of peritoneal dialysis, continuous ambulatory peritoneal dialysis (CAPD) (Drukker, 1983a). The simple machine-free method, which required the manual exchange of four to five bags of dialysate per day, allowed patients greater mobility and freedom from the artificial kidney machine (Drukker, 1983a). The continuous nature of the dialysis also enabled many more patients, including the elderly and those with diabetes, to be treated safely in the home (Stason & Barnes, 1985). CAPD quickly surpassed hemodialysis as the most popular form of home therapy, with more than twice as many patients currently receiving CAPD as home hemodialysis (9,995 compared to 4,125 in 1984).[12]

Federal payment policy may have contributed inadvertently to the decline in the proportion of patients on home hemodialysis, but it was not the only influence on choice of therapy. Patients undergoing dialysis today are on average older and sicker than those treated prior to the 1972 legislation (Rubin, 1984; Eggers, Connerton & McMullan, 1984). Some physicians believe that most of these patients are not suitable candidates for home dialysis because of either their health or living conditions. It must also be noted that many patients receiving dialysis in the early 1970s before the advent of public insurance underwent home care out of financial necessity, not because they desired it. When given the choice, many patients elect center dialysis, which offers nursing support and social interaction as well as the basic treatment. The ESRD experience illustrates that reimbursement policy is but one of several factors and perhaps not the most important in determining the use of different therapies and treatment settings.

RATE REDUCTION

A potential advantage of prospective payment lies in the fact that once efficiency improvements have been made, the government can share in the savings by lowering per-treatment rates. In theory, the "ratcheting down" of rates should occur frequently enough that government continually shares in the cost savings (Vladeck, 1982). However, the federal government did not lower facility rates for over a decade despite evidence that substantial reductions had been made in the costs of dialysis therapy. Although BHI officials considered the screen on facility reimbursement to be a temporary measure, they did not act to readjust the rates until forced to do so by Congress (Rettig, 1982). It was not until the adoption of the 1978 end-stage renal disease amendments that Congress formally endorsed the program's use of prospective payment and provided the Health Care Financing Administration (HCFA), the successor to the Bureau of Health

Insurance, with guidelines for lowering the fixed fees per treatment. The amendments specified that facility rates should be established on a cost-related basis and designed with incentives for encouraging more cost-effective delivery of dialysis services (Federal Register, 1983).

HCFA subsequently conducted audits of 38 freestanding facilities and 67 hospitals to determine whether rate reductions were indeed feasible (Kusserow, 1982). Remarkably, HCFA officials had not had legislative authority to require facilities to provide them with cost data prior to the 1978 amendments. From its survey of dialysis providers, HCFA estimated the median cost per treatment at $108 for freestanding facilities and $135 for hospital-based facilities (Davis, 1982). Freestanding facilities operating at the median level earned a $30 profit on each session. The vast majority of hospitals had applied for exceptions to the cost screen and were being reimbursed an average of $159 per treatment and thus retained a surplus of $24 per treatment. The difference between audited costs for independent and hospital facilities reflected, in part, HCFA's policy of routinely granting exemptions to hospitals (Rettig, 1982).

In May 1981, HCFA proposed a single rate based on the audit data for independent facilities. The rate would be set at $130 per treatment, or 120% of the median costs for the freestanding facilities (Rettig, 1982). Proprietary facilities and the Office of Management and Budget had called for a single rate to promote competition between freestanding and hospital facilities. Under a single rate, hospitals would either reduce their costs or patients would of necessity be shifted to less-expensive independent facilities. Congress resisted this proposal because of concerns that hospitals would be driven from the marketplace with a single lower rate (U.S. Congress, Senate, 1982a, 19–20). Instead, in the 1981 Omnibus Budget Reconciliation Act (OBRA), Congress mandated a dual-rate payment system, one rate for hospitals and a lower rate for freestanding facilities. The dual rates were designed to maintain hospitals in the dialysis business in spite of their higher costs. Moreover, Congress recognized that hospital facilities were more likely than independents to propose transplants or place patients on home care. To encourage home dialysis further, Congress advocated a composite rate for home and facilities that would in effect provide facilities with a "rent" for either initiating or transferring patients to home care (Romeo, 1984).

Regulations establishing a dual composite rate and reducing dialysis payments were issued in November 1982 (Romeo, 1984). But opposition to lower dialysis rates and HCFA's use of a questionable statistical methodology in computing facility payments delayed their implementation until August 1983. The General Accounting Office criticized HCFA for not validating the cost data reported to fiscal intermediaries; others pointed out the arithmetic errors made in the calculations of the rates (Kusserow, 1982; Federal Register, 1983). Critics charged that the rates resulted more from an assessment of what was politically feasible rather than from an unbiased analysis of the cost data (Federal Register, 1983).

HCFA's response to its congressional mandate illustrates the analytical complexity and the political compromises inherent in rate setting. By law, the agency was required to examine alternative approaches to rate setting, but HCFA did not choose the methodology that would yield the greatest savings for the government (Federal Register, 1983). Instead, it decided to average the costs of hospital and freestanding facilities as a basis for rate setting, and then make minor adjustments in the hospital rates (U.S. Congress, Senate, 1982a). Had HCFA decreased the fixed prices for hospitals and freestanding facilities proportionately, it would have generated greater program savings. The General Accounting Office argued that HCFA was in effect providing windfall profits to freestanding facilities (U.S. Congress, Senate, 1982a). HCFA defended its methodology on the grounds that the proportionate rate reductions would have penalized the more-efficient freestanding facilities (Federal Register, 1983).

The average composite rates that finally went into effect on August 1, 1983 were $131 per dialysis treatment for hospital-based and $127 for freestanding facilities (Eggers, 1984). (HCFA had based the fees on a formula that took into account the distribution of patients treated in the home and at facilities.) The rates would be allowed to vary to reflect local labor costs from a low of $114 to a high of $148 for hospitals and from $109 to $143 for freestanding facilities. Although HCFA maintained an exemption process for facilities with justifiably higher costs, it tightened up criteria for allowing exemptions (Federal Register, 1983).

HCFA sought other program savings by reducing the level of the monthly payments to physicians (Federal Register, 1983). Although the monthly capitation rate for physicians had remained nearly constant since 1974, a widespread perception existed that many renal physicians had profited excessively from the publicly funded program. In congressional hearings on prospective reimbursement for dialysis services, several senators denounced a treatment center that purchased five Mercedes-Benzes—one for each physician working in the facility (U.S. Congress, Senate, 1982b).[13] The visibility of renal physicians' incomes and fringe benefits gave HCFA the political support necessary to reduce the monthly capitation rates from an average of $220 to $184 per patient.[14] The monthly retainer was applied to both facility and home patients. The composite rate was designed to remove any financial disincentives in payment policy so that physicians would place patients on home dialysis whenever it was considered medically appropriate. HCFA might have proposed even lower physician payments, but was constrained by fears that doctors would cut back on the services provided to renal patients if the reductions were too large (Federal Register, 1983).

Some of the short-term effects of the lower rates can already be judged. For the first time in the ESRD program's history, total reimbursements in 1984 actually declined, despite a substantial increase in patient enrollments. Reimbursements on per-patient basis decreased by nearly 19% from $24,800 to $20,200 (HCFA, 1984). More stringent criteria all but eliminated hospital facilities' use of the exception process; only 13 facilities escaped from the fixed-payment system in 1984.[15] Neither the composite facility rate nor the revised rules for physician payment have influenced the percentage of patients receiving home hemodialysis. The number of patients undergoing home hemodialysis in 1984 is lower than that in 1980 (4,125 vs. 4,715)(HCFA, 1984). In contrast, CAPD continues to grow in popularity. Despite the reductions in payment, large numbers of hospitals have not withdrawn from the business of providing dialysis services (Federal Register, 1986).

CONCLUSIONS

Inelegantly executed though it was, the ESRD program's prospective-payment strategy saved the federal government money. The fixed price per outpatient treatment constrained the growth in total program expenditures. At the same time the ESRD payment methods provided dialysis facilities with a strong motivation to reduce their labor and materials costs. While the price of dialysis services remained constant for more than a decade, the payments for other Medicare services increased dramatically. For example, the reimbursement per enrollee for disabled individuals eligible for Medicare increased from $344 in 1974 to $941 in 1980. Had dialysis reimbursements escalated at the same rate, they would have expanded from approximately $23,000 per patient per year in 1974 to more than $64,000 in 1980. Even with high inflation in unregulated services such as inpatient dialysis and transplantation, the rate of increase in ESRD expenditures was far less than that for other parts of the Medicare program.

Although the per-patient costs of dialysis treatment have declined dramatically, the government did not benefit as much as it could have had the program been more effectively managed. Medicare's establishment of a generous $150 fee per treatment was understandable given the initial need both to ensure an adequate supply of facilities and to accommodate differently situated providers. When evidence of cost savings in dialysis therapy became available, the ESRD program should, however, have decreased the rates. In fact, Medicare officials only reduced the rates when confronted with congressional pressure. The ESRD program's loose administration of the exception system, in which it routinely granted hospitals' requests for a waiver of the $150 fee, was another source of inefficiency. By its failure to readjust the rates and to apply them uniformly to hospital-based and independent facilities, the federal government potentially sacrificed millions of dollars in cost savings. A significant portion of the benefits from prospective payment thus accrued to dialysis providers and not to the government.

The federal government's failings in rate setting can be attributed, at least in part, to the small size of the ESRD program relative to the larger Medicare program (Sadler, 1981). Although a program with nearly a $2 billion yearly budget, the expenditures on ESRD accounted for less than 3.7% of the total Medicare budget in 1983. Congress and senior administrative officials undoubtedly placed priority on those items in the Medicare budget that would have more substantial budgetary implications.[16] Even if officials were to cut ESRD expenditures by half—a political impossibility—these cost savings would amount to less than 2% of the total Medicare budget.

The weaknesses in ESRD program management reflect structural characteristics of federal programs generally (Rettig, 1982). Early in its history, the ESRD program was considered a possible prototype for other health insurance initiatives. As a consequence, senior administrative officials and congressional staff devoted substantial effort to devising an innovative reimbursement policy. Once the initial payment mechanisms were established, the program fell victim to management neglect. Like other federal programs, the ESRD program was disrupted by periodic reorganizations, competition among bureaus for policy and operational authority, and frequent turnover of senior staff (Demkovich, 1980).[17] Discontinuities in staff and leadership led to delays and inconsistencies in reimbursement policy.

Still other problems in rate setting resulted from the ESRD program's lack of experience with prospective payment. Prospective payment requires a different mix of management skills than retrospective cost-based reimbursement; the government must act as a prudent regulator/buyer rather than a payer of health services. At a minimum, prospective payment requires the acquisition of large amounts of data and the ability to negotiate with hospitals and physicians. Medicare's expertise, however, lay in claims processing and the accounting principles of cost-plus reimbursement. When administrative officials encountered obstacles in the application of prospective payment, they naturally retreated to the more familiar routines of the cost-based reimbursement system.

Throughout the ESRD program's history, the federal government experienced difficulties in the collection and analysis of the data necessary for rate setting. The ESRD program never established a regular means of collecting cost and clinical data on dialysis treatment. Nor did dialysis facilities readily provide the government with data from their financial records. Without adequate information, government regulators found it hard to determine what was either a reasonable cost or "profit" for dialysis services. Perhaps even more importantly, rate-setting methodologies were not systematically designed before data collection but devised in an ad hoc manner after the fact.

Medicare was no more successful in negotiating with health providers and overcoming the political obstacles to rate setting than it was in data collection. Government officials were not willing to pressure dialysis facilities financially. Thus rates were set at a level reflecting the costs of only moderately efficient facilities. In lowering the fees in 1983, HCFA, for example, had the opportunity to base the rates on the operating costs of a typical freestanding facility. Instead, it chose to average the costs of all freestanding and hospital-based facilities. At the urging of hospitals, Congress supported an even more generous rate-setting methodology. Neither administrative nor elected officials were willing to use the payment system to force patients into home care or independent facilities—the most cost-effective treatment settings. Cost control objectives were continually compromised in order to preserve maximum clinical freedom and patient autonomy (Rettig, 1980).

The ESRD experience illustrates some of both the opportunities and dilemmas that Medicare will confront with the implementation of prospective payment. Indeed, the methods initiated in 1973 to reimburse for kidney disease resemble those in Medicare's new payment system for inpatient hospital care; in the former, Medicare established a fixed fee per treatment session; in the latter, it relies on a fixed fee per case. The ESRD program demonstrates the potential of prospective payment to encourage the adoption of cost-saving technology and the use of less-expensive treatment settings. Medicare's prospective payment system may also resemble the ESRD program by creating a motivation to reduce the length of treatment or stay. The economic incentives in the new payment system might, however, be diminished because the fixed fees apply only to Medicare beneficiaries. The effects of the payment incentives could be reduced further by the fact that Medicare continues to pay physicians on a fee-for-service basis. Under a fee-for-service system, physicians might offset any facility savings by increasing the volume of services provided to patients.

Although the control of Medicare expenditures is currently a major budgetary priority, the Medicare program may confront management problems in rate setting that are similar to those faced by the ESRD program. The Medicare system will likely have difficulty recruiting and retaining the staff required to implement a highly complex regulatory system. Staffing problems will be exacerbated by frequent government reorganizations and changes in elected officials. In turn, this organizational disarray may prevent the necessary data acquisition. If Medicare experienced severe problems in establishing a rate-setting methodology for a single disease, one can imagine the difficulties the program will confront in the administration of a payment system based on 467 separate diagnosis-related groups.

Medicare can undoubtedly anticipate increasing efforts to manipulate payment policy to promote the use of specific therapies and treatment settings. In the payment system for ESRD, physician groups and for-profit facilities attempted to shape reimbursement policy to achieve their economic or clinical objectives. Advocates of CAPD, home hemodialysis, center dialysis, and transplantation each took their special claims for payment to Congress and rate-setting officials. Under prospective payment, government officials will increasingly be called upon to mediate clinical disputes among proponents of different therapies and institutions. Teaching hospitals may, for example, lobby rate setters to raise their payments relative to community hospitals.[18]

Because of the potential dilemmas in managing prospective payment, the federal government may need to combine it with other payment methods to achieve more substantial savings. Several commentators have suggested that the use of competitive contracting might improve the efficiency of the dialysis program (Stason & Barnes, 1985). Instead of allowing dialysis suppliers to charge widely varying prices to individuals and facilities, HCFA could negotiate a fixed price for suppliers that would apply to patients located throughout the country. Similarly, Medicare could negotiate fixed-price contracts with health care providers such as health maintenance organizations and preferred provider organizations. Although prospective payment represents the first step towards the federal government's effective use of its enormous market power, Medicare still has a long way to go to become a prudent regulator and buyer of health services.

NOTES

1. Personal interview with James Mongan, M.D., former professional staff member, U.S. Senate, Committee on Finance.

2. Per Mongan interview, discussions of alternative payment methods predate the 1972 Social Security amendments. See, for example, Feldstein, 1966.

3. Per Mongan interview.

4. Personal interview with Irwin Wolkstein, formerly a senior official, Bureau of Health Insurance, Social Security Administration.

5. Per Wolkstein interview.

6. Per Wolkstein interview.

7. Although the majority of hospitals received exceptions to the cost screen, few freestanding facilities were granted exceptions. The freestanding facilities were for the most part investor owned.

8. In our interviews, some dialysis facilities reported dialysis times as short as two hours per session.

9. Personal interview with Mariane Alter, Centers for Disease Control. Data on reuse is from the Centers for Disease Control's Hepatitis Survey. The percentage of patients practicing reuse may actually approach 80% as large facilities are more likely to practice reuse than are small facilities.

10. Manufacturers report that the demand for new dialyzers has continued to drop since 1983.

11. In an interview, Edward Berger of National Medical Care suggested that manufacturers of dialyzers had a major incentive to reduce manufacturing costs and dialyzer prices in order to discourage reuse. An official of Baxter Travenol attributed the drop in dialyzer prices to reuse, competition, and automation.

12. Unpublished data from HCFA.

13. After the rate reductions, the General Accounting Office issued a report that found that the degree of physician involvement with patients had been overestimated and that physician fees should be lowered accordingly. See U.S. General Accounting Office, "Changes Needed in Medicare Payments to Physicians Under the End Stage Renal Disease Program," GAO/HRD-85-14, February 1985.

14. In 1978, Christopher Blagg noted that the capitation method of physician payment increased the political visibility of nephrologists' incomes. Congress had expressed dismay in the level of physician payments as early as 1976.

15. Interview with an official of the Health Care Financing Administration.

16. Per Mongan interview.

17. See also Rettig and Marks, 1982, for a discussion of the administrative problems

confronting ESRD reimbursement policy. For a more general discussion of the problems that governments face with prospective payment, see Sapolsky et al., 1987.

18. The new Prospective Payment Assessment Commission (ProPAC) is already confronting similar pressures from health institutions.

12

Medical Technology Meets DRGs: Acquiring Magnetic Resonance Imaging under Prospective Payment

John R. Kimberly, Laura E. Roper, Scott D. Ramsey, Alan L. Hillman, and J. Sanford Schwartz

Medical technology has been argued by some to be "the culprit behind health care costs," in part due to its overutilization (Altman & Blendon, 1979; Maloney & Rogers, 1979). At least part of this problem has been attributed to the fee-for-service payment system (Newhouse, 1978) where providers are reimbursed retrospectively for each service performed. Fee-for-service payment assures providers of income from the use of expensive technology, whether or not a patient derives significant benefit from the procedure, and thus significantly limits financial risk from investment in new technologies.

In the early 1970s, concern heightened over technology's contribution to medical inflation. One response to this concern was federal authorization for state implementation of certificate-of-need (CON) laws. As part of the National Health Planning and Resources Development Act (PL 93–641), each state's CON regulations required health care facilities to submit an application for approval from the regional health planning agency before undertaking major investments in new medical facilities and equipment. Later in the decade, many researchers and policymakers began to question the effectiveness of CON, as evidence began to mount that the program did little to slow the acquisition of technology or ease the spiraling pace of medical inflation (Sloan, 1981; Salkever & Bice, 1976).

In 1983, the federal government implemented the Prospective Payment System (PPS) for Medicare hospital inpatients. By giving hospitals a fixed payment per admission, PPS provides hospitals with a financial incentive to operate more efficiently and, presumably, to consider more carefully the costs and benefits of investments in new technology. When PPS was enacted, reimbursement for the purchase of capital and medical equipment was not included in the diagnosis-related group (DRG) classification system, although specific provisions in the new law mandated feasibility studies for "folding" capital into the DRG payment rate. Thus, hospitals continued to be reimbursed for new building and equipment on a retrospective, "reasonable cost" basis. Although there is evidence that PPS has reduced hospital costs (Guterman & Dobson, 1986), it remains unclear (in part as a result of the capital exemption clause) whether more "prudent" use of new medical technology has been a factor in the savings.

Given the intended goals of PPS, we examined the diffusion of magnetic resonance imaging (MRI), an expensive new diagnostic technology that became commercially available just prior to the passage of PPS. Three key questions we addressed were: (1) How, if at all, has PPS affected hospitals' decisions to acquire MRI? (2) How have changes in the reimbursement environment (including PPS) and in the nature of competition in local markets influenced patterns of ownership and siting of MRI, particularly in comparison to computerized tomography (CT), an expensive diagnostic technology introduced prior to PPS? and (3) What does MRI, as a prototype high-cost, equipment-embodied medical innovation in the post-PPS era, signal for the changes that are likely to occur in the adoption and diffusion of other new medical technologies in the future?

To answer these questions, a multidisciplinary research team at the Leonard Davis Institute of Health Economics at the University of Pennsylvania has been conducting a study of MRI diffusion consisting of: (1) a multivariate analysis of hospital adoption of MRI using American Hospital Association (AHA) data, Area Resource File (ARF) data, and data on MRI ownership gathered at the University of Pennsylvania; (2) a national survey of senior executives at hospitals and freestanding imaging organizations (FIOs) that have invested in MRI and a sample of hospitals and freestanding imaging organizations (FIOs) which have not,[1] and; (3) case studies, conducted in four cities, of decision-making about MRI acquisition in both hospitals and FIOs. The research thus addresses the diffusion process at two levels, organization and market. At the organizational level (either hospital or FIO), we were concerned with discovering those factors that affect the decision to acquire or not to acquire an MRI unit. At the level of the market area, we were interested in explaining the extent, timing, and pattern of diffusion.

The advantage of the overall research design is that the results of each part can verify, complement, expand, or otherwise inform the results of the other parts. The multivariate analysis covers all 6,000 acute care hospitals in the United States, focusing on the attributes of the hospitals themselves and their immediate environments as predictors of adoption. The survey of senior executives at hospitals and FIOs focuses on the decision-making process in their institutions, and targets perceptions about the health care environment, MRI technology, and where that technology fits into the overall strategies their institutions are pursuing. All adopting organizations and a stratified random sample of nonadopting insti-

tutions are being surveyed. The case studies explore in greater depth the acquisition decision process and are based on interviews with hospital CEOs, CFOs,
chiefs of the medical staff, chiefs of radiology, board chairpersons, and directors
of freestanding sites. The multivariate analyses examine a number of attributes
of hospitals and markets that may be associated with and influence technology
acquisition decisions. The survey focuses on the decision-making process and
at least one key decision maker's perceptions of the role of many of those
"objective" factors. The case studies provide more detail about these factors,
help interpret the findings from the other two parts, and generate broader insights
into the decision process *per se*.

This chapter combines data collected on patterns of ownership and siting
nationally with insights from the case studies to begin to answer the question of
how technology acquisition decisions have been influenced by PPS. The first
section briefly summarizes national data on the rate and pattern of diffusion of
MRI. In the second section we go beyond this statistical portrait and, using data
from the case studies, explore how changes in the health care environment have
affected decision-making about investment in MRI.

MACRO EFFECTS: MRI DIFFUSION 1981–1986

MRI first became available commercially in 1981, when the FDA approved
several manufacturers' units for sale outside research institutions. A graph of
the growth in numbers of units installed since that time would exhibit the typical
sigmoid-shaped diffusion pattern associated with successful innovations. Between 1981 and December 1986, approximately 550 units were installed across
the United States, with the largest increase in installations occurring between
1984 and 1985. By the end of 1986, significantly, slightly more than half of
these units were not located on hospital grounds. In contrast, only 19% of CT
units were installed outside of hospitals during the first four years of its clinical
availability (Hillman & Schwartz, 1985). Of the MRI units *not* located on hospital
grounds, 60% were in FIOs. The rest of the non-hospital-based MRI units were
"mobile"; that is, installed in trailers that traveled to multiple health care centers
under a variety of contractual arrangements.

Between 1981 and 1983, MRI adoption occurred primarily in large hospitals
having research and teaching affiliations. A majority of these early MRI units
were installed at hospitals with more than 500 beds; almost three-fourths of them
were located in institutions with more than 400 beds. The majority of units at
these large medical centers were purchased outright by the hospital, in part
because of their access to capital and in part because of attractive financial
managements provided by the manufacturers.

Beginning in 1984, the number of MRI units located off hospital grounds
grew rapidly, and in 1985 the number of mobile units increased significantly as
well. The sources involved in financing non-hospital-based units are diverse and
growing. They include physician groups, intermediaries that set up MRI sites,

MRI manufacturers, other investors, and even hospitals themselves. A small but significant number of FIOs and mobile units (about 3%) have been financed through multihospital consortia. The mobile scanners travel among the hospitals of the consortium; FIOs are placed at a strategic site readily accessible to patients and the financing institutions.

From 1985 to 1986, many MRI units were acquired by smaller hospitals (under 400 beds). The diversity in financing for this "wave" of acquisitions was much greater than for the initial group of hospital investors. From 1985 to 1986, hospitals increasingly used leasing and joint ventures with physicians and others to acquire MRI units. Leasing was used to finance about 20% of MRI scanners during this period, regardless of where they were sited or who operated them. The number of operational mobile units also continued to expand rapidly. By 1986, mobile MRI scanners accounted for approximately 25% of all MRI units installed in the United States.

In sum, diversity in siting and complexity of ownership characterized the first five years of significant growth in MRI. The majority of MRI units installed by the end of 1986 were at least partially owned by hospitals. In cases where the hospital was not the sole owner of an MRI unit, the most likely partners in financing were physicians, yet many hospitals established units with other investors also. Over one-half of all MRI units were not installed in hospitals, a significant change from early CT diffusion, where less than one-fifth of early units were sited off hospital grounds. A significant number of mobile units became operational. Leasing, either from the manufacturers themselves or from intermediaries designed to set up MRI sites, became an increasingly common vehicle for financing acquisition of MRI scanners by the end of 1986.

MICRO EFFECTS: INFLUENCES ON THE DECISION-MAKING PROCESS

The emerging trends in siting and ownership noted in the previous section were undoubtedly influenced by changes in the health care environment during the mid–1980s—an environment characterized by the introduction of PPS and by a number of other forces converging to increase the levels of competition between hospitals in local market areas. The evolving health environment during this time created uncertainty in many areas—uncertainty that has diminished in some respects with the passage of time but that has shaped patterns of institutional response. In this section of the chapter, our aim is to breathe some life into the statistical portrait by reporting on how the decision makers themselves described the MRI decision process. Our interviews revealed a number of important uncertainties confronting decision makers at the organizational level. These uncertainties, in turn, influenced the hospital decision-making process and led, ultimately, to one of three outcomes.

Uncertainties at the Organizational Level

MRI created uncertainty for managers on several fronts. The likelihood and level of insurance reimbursement for MRI scans was far from clear when the technology was first introduced. Prior to November 1985, Medicare did not designate MRI as a covered service, and many private insurers paid for MRI scans on a "case-by-case" basis, if at all. In addition, MRI was initially seen to offer few clinical advantages over other diagnostic technologies (advantages were primarily in imaging the brain). Thus, many managers were unsure whether MRI would emerge as a replacement for other established diagnostic technologies (in particular computerized tomography [CT]) or would simply complement the hospital's existing diagnostic armamentarium.

The regulatory environment on both the federal and state level was also of little help in assuaging managers' doubts about the prudence of investing in MRI. Many states, concerned that MRI was not a proven "need" to the community, established tight regional limits on the number of MRI units that would be granted a certificate of need, a strategy that virtually precluded siting of units outside of major research and teaching hospitals in these areas (Steinberg & Cohen, 1984). As a result, many hospitals desiring MRI could not become involved in the purchase or siting of units. Some states even controlled the installation of MRIs in FIOs, regardless of whether a hospital was or was not involved in the unit's financing and operation.

The Prospective Payment System itself represented an important source of uncertainty, since few managers knew in 1983 how this new method of reimbursement for Medicare inpatients would affect hospital profits. Although hospitals in fact achieved record profits during the first two years of PPS, this did not change the fact that prospective payment turned the incentives for patient care upside down, because now *reducing* the number of tests and procedures performed on patients would increase hospital profits. In this light, MRI was not attractive since it initially seemed to be merely an "add-on" innovation rather than a technology that could replace other expensive diagnostic tests.

Aside from the uncertainty generated by the new Prospective Payment System, there were long delays in determining such key federal policies as support for medical residents and continuing federal support for state health systems agencies (HSAs). In addition, at the time PPS was passed in Congress, studies were mandated to explore the possibility of folding payments for capital and equipment into the DRG payment system, a possibility that struck terror into the fiscal minds of many hospital administrators, particularly those with aging facilities and equipment. Managers could not anticipate how the resolution of these policies affected their institutions' financial situation, which in turn affected the priorities placed on acquiring new technology versus other hospital objectives.

The federal government added to the complexity of managerial decision-making regarding MRI in the spring of 1986 when Congress proposed several major changes in the tax code for individuals and businesses. Of particular interest were proposals to eliminate the investment tax credit and lengthen the depreciation schedules for capital and equipment, since such measures would significantly reduce the financial attractiveness of MRI to investors. Concern about these financial factors was displayed in managers' investment decisions, for the rate of increase in newly operated MRI units slowed significantly in 1986 compared to the two previous years.

PPS, among other factors, was changing the relationship between the hospital administration and staff physicians. DRGs encouraged hospital administrators to become more involved in physicians' practices, since by encouraging doctors' efficiency in patient care, hospitals could increase their net revenues. Managers were also aware, however, that physicians saw this involvement as a threat both to their autonomy as patients' advocates and to the financially beneficial relationship they enjoyed with hospitals. Technology played an important role in this dynamic since physicians tend to regard acquiring the most-advanced medical technology as an important aspect of maintaining quality patient care.

These issues played out in three ways in the case of MRI. First, administrators recognized that the way they dealt with MRI would set a precedent for future hospital-physician interactions, particularly joint ventures. They thus had to weigh the benefits of working with a certain number of physicians through an MRI joint venture with the risk that this would lead other doctors to expect similar cooperation with their requests for new technologies. Many of these future requests, administrators postulated, would include projects that were inconsistent with the financial means or the goals of the hospital. Second, administrators were concerned with the loss of control inherent in a joint venture. Third, although many doctors were ''offering'' to finance MRI partially or fully themselves, approving such ventures entailed serious unresolved legal and ethical issues regarding the potential for conflict of interest from these units. If physician-financing of MRI came to be defined as inappropriate, it could damage the hospital's image in the community and create serious (and expensive) legal difficulties as well.

Finally, the MRI manufacturers themselves were creating uncertainty for hospital managers considering purchase of a scanner. By 1984, no fewer than 10 separate companies were producing MRI units. Rumors of potential mergers and bankruptcies among these manufacturers were widespread. Decision makers had to choose from a wide array of models and several important features, including field strength (ranging from 0.15-tesla to 2.0-tesla magnets), magnet type (superconducting, permanent, or resistive), and alternative computer software systems—each having enormous implications for cost, possibilities for siting, and range of medical applications afforded. In addition, the prior experience many administrators had with having to purchase several generations of CT scanners made them think twice about purchasing a unit that might become ''obsolete'' in a year or two. Lastly, the possibility that a unit would be purchased just in time for the manufacturer to go bankrupt or merge with another company (resulting in lost software support and maintenance) loomed large in many managers' minds.

In sum, a host of conditions, many of which did not exist prior to the imposition of PPS or were altered with the new law, increased the financial risks associated with purchase of MRI. Changes in government laws and regulations, hospital-physician dynamics, and characteristics of the technology itself increased uncertainty in a number of areas. Adding to the complexity of the decision-making process, however, was the "promise" MRI held for hospitals hoping to improve their market position in an increasingly competitive health care environment.

The Promise of MRI

Why would managers want to acquire MRI? While many of the above-mentioned factors contributed to delayed acquisition of MRI, PPS had another important consequence—it intensified competition among health care providers. PPS did this in three ways. First, by making hospitals assume the financial risk of Medicare inpatient care, PPS intensified competition for patients covered by traditional, retrospectively reimbursing private insurance. Second, since Medicare continued to pay for outpatient services on a retrospective, reasonable-cost basis after DRGs were implemented, hospital outpatient treatment became a more financially desirable alternative for Medicare patients who could receive such care. Third, it quickly became known to administrators that some DRGs were money makers while others were financial losers. By working to attract Medicare patients who were likely to fall into a "profitable" DRG, a hospital could improve its financial position. Finally, since many of a hospital's costs are fixed (at least in the short run), high admission rates were important to increase hospital profits. In this way, competition for all patients increased.

In light of these changes brought about by PPS, MRI presented an opportunity for hospitals and private physicians to expand their patient base and remain competitive. By enhancing the image of an institution, technology may attract patients and doctors to that hospital. Indeed, the acquisition of hospital-based and non-hospital-based technology became an important component of many hospitals' strategic plans to achieve a competitive edge in the community (Whitcomb, 1988). Under such circumstances, a highly promising, state-of-the-art, noninvasive diagnostic technology that would be competitive with CT scanning and could be established in an outpatient setting generated a lot of interest. The question posed to potential adopters was how to enjoy the benefits of the technology while minimizing the financial risks.

Some of the uncertainties noted above have arisen since the implementation of PPS; others accompany the introduction of any expensive new technology in medicine. Our field interviews revealed a heightened complexity in the investment decision-making process, characterized by the involvement of a large number of individuals and parties, resulting in a multiplicity of ownership and financing arrangements. Process and outcome were also shaped by environmental factors that were unique to each of the regions studied. Through our case studies we identified several important trends that we postulate may represent new patterns of decision-making in the post-PPS health care environment.

PATTERNS OF DECISION-MAKING AT THE HOSPITAL LEVEL

To determine how hospitals and individuals perceived the opportunities and constraints in the health care environment and how those perceptions affected their MRI investment decisions, we conducted a series of in-depth interviews in the summer and fall of 1987 in four metropolitan regions—one each in the east, midwest, south, and southwest United States. The cities selected (including the contiguous suburban areas) were chosen for their regional distribution, for their distinctive regulatory environments, and for a range in health care market size. For the purpose of anonymity these cities will hereafter be referred to as Sunnydale (southwest), Prairie City (midwest), Belle City (south), and Metropolis (east).

All of the areas studied had at least one medical school and at least one teaching hospital. Each city had several operational MRI units, although the mix of ownership and the predominance of hospital-based versus freestanding units varied among regions. Of the units in Prairie City, 75% were fully owned or leased by hospitals; no units were located off hospital grounds. In contrast, none of the units in Sunnydale was fully hospital owned, and only 1 was leased by a hospital. However, all but 1 of these units were located at a hospital. Belle City had 4 MRI units at the time of our interviews, 3 of which were located on hospital grounds. Two units were owned solely by a hospital; the other 2 were financed in whole or in part through physician investment. Finally, Metropolis, a large urban center, had 14 units located in the area. Half of these units were at least partially owned by nonhospital investors. Six units were located off hospital grounds. Our objectives in the interviews were to determine the kinds of factors that influenced decision-making about MRI and to identify, where possible, patterns—across locations and/or across markets—in decision processes and outcomes.

Factors in the Decision Process

In all four communities, hospital administration respondents expressed a preference to be sole owners of a unit if that were feasible. When asked why they desired sole ownership, the most common responses were that they wished to avoid legal questions regarding profit versus not-for-profit status of the site, conflict-of-interest problems arising from physician investment, and the precedent-setting problem of allowing doctors to use hospitals for their own entrepreneurial ventures. These reasons often came under the general statement that hospital administration wished to retain "control" of MRI.

Ultimately, however, hospitals had to weigh their desire to own and control the technology against the hospital's overall strategy, the cost and potential profitability of a unit, and competitive pressures. Hospital administrators clearly were aware of the financial risks associated with investing in a technology that was very expensive to purchase and to maintain. At the same time, competitive pressures clearly motivated administrators, even in smaller community hospitals, seriously to consider acquiring a unit. The administrator of an 80-bed hospital in Sunnydale allowed a staff physician to set up an MRI center on hospital grounds for "PR advantages" and with the hope that neurologists from other hospitals would put more of their patients in the hospital. Pressures were particularly keen when a competing hospital had acquired or had plans to acquire a unit (either alone or in conjunction with a physician group), or when an intermediary group, attached to no one hospital, was considering opening a nearby outpatient MRI facility.

Often, hospitals that did not consider themselves high-tech hospitals deferred the decision to acquire an MRI. One interesting reason given by some hospitals for not adopting MRI was that it would merely discover diseases requiring referral to tertiary hospitals, resulting in loss of revenue from those patients. Thus, these smaller hospitals often accepted the risks of allowing the "big boys" to have the MRI scanners. However, many of these same institutions would subsequently be moved to action upon hearing that a hospital they perceived as a competitor began plans to acquire a unit, or if the hospital's own radiology and/or neurology staff decided to purchase one.

Bunching was common; that is, once one unit became operational, several more units entered the market within the next 6 to 12 months. Occasionally, administrators admitted that they acquired an MRI unit knowing that the investment would be unprofitable, but argued that they could not afford not to have one. Large tertiary hospitals often saw MRI (and other advanced technologies) as central to maintaining their image as a leader in high-technology services. One hospital administrator in Prairie City called his staff doctors to see if they were interested in having medical technologies he saw on the evening news. Other cited widespread physician support for MRI and did not want to risk deterioration of hospital-medical staff relations by refusing to acquire a unit. Often, units perceived by administration as potential financial losers were acquired through leasing arrangements and joint ventures, thereby minimizing the financial risks.

Deciding that acquisition is desirable (or conversely, that acquisition should be deferred) is often only one of the early steps in the decision-making process. Faced with the high cost of the technology, an uncertain health care environment, and competitive pressures, potential adopters wanted to identify and exploit all the available opportunities afforded by MRI while avoiding undue financial risk. We found that decision processes varied widely but resulted in one of three outcomes: the hospital-centered purchase, the physician-hospital contract, or the physician-centered purchase.

Decision Outcomes

The Hospital-Centered Purchase

Aside from the major teaching hospitals, a large number of hospitals that purchased their own units were major tertiary care centers that regarded themselves as technology leaders in their communities. Although discussion about MRI was often initiated by physicians, occasionally a member of the administration or the hospital board first raised the possibility of acquisition. A formal decision to acquire the technology tended to be made rapidly, but actual purchase was often delayed, in part due to concerns about profitability and in part because of uncertainty in choosing the best manufacturer and model of scanner to assure the highest return. If CON approval was sought, additional delays of up to one year were common. This was a delay many institutions were willing to suffer, however, to ensure control of the unit, as mentioned above.

Often, hospital acquisition decisions were a response to the administration's knowledge that radiologists at the hospital were exploring the possibility of setting up a freestanding site. A typical scenario was as follows: the head of radiology learns of MRI at a scientific meeting and approaches the hospital administration with the proposal that the hospital should have a unit. Management balks at the $1–2 million price tag, but does not rule out the possibility of acquisition at a later date. At this point the radiologist invites an intermediary into the picture, who in turn organizes a presentation (not always known to or attended by administration) showing the merits of its MRI startup program. When the administration learns of the situation with the intermediaries (and the radiologists' apparent resolve to acquire MRI), their attitude softens, and ways are found to finance a unit. Thus, ironically, intermediaries were often used to force the *hospital* into purchasing a scanner, rather than serving as a viable financing alternative for acquiring the technology. Thus, the "traditional" hospital-centered purchase at times resulted from a decidedly nontraditional negotiating process.

An increasingly popular MRI acquisition option for hospitals is the leasing of units from intermediaries. This option is particularly attractive for smaller and intermediate-sized hospitals (fewer than 400 beds) that simply do not have the patient base or the financial and personnel resources to purchase and maintain a unit. Because there were so many intermediaries in operation, many of which were trying to break into new markets, hospitals could shop around for the best deal. For many hospitals, the intermediary provides a particularly low-cost way to gain access to large, expensive, superconducting magnets. Manufacturers, in turn, like dealing with the intermediaries because of their experience with MRI and because it avoids involvement in hospital infighting. Finally, the risk to the intermediaries is fairly low, especially to those that specialize in mobile units.

Intermediaries can line up a dozen customers on the route of one mobile unit. If a given hospital is not generating enough customers to justify the hours the unit is spending at the site, it is a small matter to reduce the hours and spend more time at another, more productive site. As the popularity of this arrangement grows, intermediaries have indicated that their clientele is not limited exclusively to the smaller hospitals (which is what they originally expected), but also consists of a mix of larger community hospitals and tertiary care centers.

The Hospital-Physician Contract

In the "hospital-physician contract," administrators and physician-investors agree to share the risk of acquiring an MRI unit. This results in one of several outcomes, including true hospital-physician joint ventures (JVs) where both parties invest in a unit located on hospital grounds; total physician-investor ownership of a unit located on hospital grounds; or hospital-physician or physician-only financing of a unit located off hospital grounds, with promotion, public relations, and other services provided by the hospital.

The process of reaching agreement often began with the scenario outlined in the hospital-centered process described above. In the "hospital-physician contract," however, the hospital agreed to relinquish some control in return for reducing its financial liabilities in undertaking the project. This outcome typically occurred in medium-sized hospitals (300–500 beds). More limited in their access to capital, these hospitals often decided to pursue a tertiary image for selected services while remaining a community hospital on the whole.

We divided the decision process into two broad strategies—the "meeting of the minds" or "jockeying for position." In both cases the process usually began as before, with physicians (most frequently radiologists) approaching the administration with a proposal that the hospital purchase a unit. In this scenario (after what may be a short or an extended process, often involving the hospital's board of trustees), the hospital made it clear that outright purchase of an MRI was impossible. Usually, the physicians' next step was to make an alternative proposal, involving some form of physician-hospital (and possibly third-party) venture.

In "the meeting of the minds," the hospital readily agreed to the physicians' proposal. The hospital's readiness to agree usually resulted from a combination of factors. In almost all cases, although the hospital's financial situation or patient base precluded outright purchase, there was a strong sense in the administration that MRI would (at least) help maintain the hospital's patient base, in particular for those patients having generous forms of third-party insurance. Of course, these hospitals did not want to lose patients to the major tertiary center(s) in town, but their apprehension increased several fold when it became known that a major rival had acquired or had plans to acquire a unit. "Meeting of the minds," therefore, often occurred in conjunction with the bunching phenomenon, so that no hospital would appear to lose its "quality" image in the community.

Other factors were important as well. In Sunnydale, for example, intense competition existed among radiologists and neurologists in the community. One doctor there, in a highly controversial move, allowed nonradiologist physicians to charge patients for reading scans at his newly installed MRI unit, thereby attracting the referrals of many neurologists from neighboring hospitals. Some hospital administrators thought that hospital-physician joint ventures were the wave of the future since they eased the pressures of raising capital and (sometimes) fostered better medical staff relations through cooperative effort towards common goals. Finally, MRI sometimes was an integral part of a new venture that the hospital wanted to undertake. This occurred in Metropolis, where one hospital wanted to start an MRI-based cancer research facility, and in Prairie City, where the goal was to establish an outpatient diagnostic center.

The other scenario, "jockeying for position," was more complicated and took various forms. In this case, the hospital was much less receptive to the idea of acquiring MRI (at least in the time frame that the physician-initiators are proposing), either through purchase, leasing, or a physician-hospital joint venture, and rejected the physicians' proposal. Administrators at the cities we visited cited several reasons why they were hesitant to acquire an MRI at their institution:

- MRI was perceived as an overpriced, underproven new medical technology. Often fueled by past experiences with CT, managers were inclined to delay purchase for several years until manufacturer viability reached a steady state, MRI became the standard of care (in the legal/liability sense), and prices fell to more reasonable levels.
- Financial difficulties at the hospital forced MRI far down the hospital's priority list. Typically, a financially troubled hospital attempted to reduce length of stay and enhance its income through diversification into outpatient services. MRI was perceived as a hindrance to achieving these goals. (Ironically, at most units we visited, outpatients accounted for up to 80% of MRI volume.)
- Hospital-physician relations were strained (in part, due to PPS), and administration was concerned that MRI could exacerbate existing tensions. Specialists, especially in the high-tech fields, often felt that the administration was not responsive to their demands, while hospital administrators frequently expressed dismay at the apparent indifference of their doctors to the budgetary constraints of the hospital. Thus, the hospital administration did not want to set a precedent by establishing a joint venture for MRI and risk further alienation of other entrepreneurial physicians (often with less meritorious proposals) expecting hospital collaboration on their projects.
- Hospital strategy was either directed to diversification (e.g., to outpatient services such as alcohol and drug abuse programs, cosmetic surgery, or anorexia and bulimia treatment programs), or was focused on a few key programs for which MRI was not essential, such as obstetrics or neonatal care.
- The hospital was concerned about the ethical and legal ramifications of joint ventures (*paranoia* was the word often used by the physicians), and thus was hesitant to undertake any such proposal. Since the hospital's financial situation precluded resolution of the problem via purchase (or leasing), physicians were left out in the cold on MRI.

In response to hospital reticence, the physicians often turned to an outside group, such as an intermediary group that set up "turnkey" operations, or a leasing company. While the hospital was unenthusiastic about MRI on the whole, the prospect of a potentially competing outpatient diagnostic radiologic facility caused them to reconsider. This reconsideration took two forms. First, there was further jockeying as the hospital tried to exert as much control as possible over the process. For example, the hospital might have agreed to put up money for the unit on the condition that it could take over negotiations with the intermediary. Hospitals also sometimes agreed to an MRI venture in return for concessions from the physicians on another issue or as part of a package deal. Physicians tended to accept these deals because their real interest was in acquiring the technology or they were unsure of the unit's profitability (early on many units were not profitable [Evens, Jost & Evans, 1985]), and thus were willing to trade off some control for reduced financial risk. The second form of reconsideration taken by the hospital resulted in undercutting the physicians by signing a leasing arrangement with a manufacturer or intermediary before the physicians concluded their own deal.

The Physician-Centered Purchase

The physician-centered purchase refers to the case where an MRI center was set up largely by doctors with little or no hospital involvement, at least in the initial acquisition. This outcome often resulted when the jockeying for position process mentioned above broke down or when physicians set off on their own, impervious to the concerns of administration. Both processes usually resulted when physicians saw administration as either indifferent or outright antagonistic to their interests. In the first case, doctors grew impatient with "the hospital bureaucracy" (in the words of one Sunnydale radiologist), and, confident of their ability to amass financial backing from other sources (usually also physicians), left the negotiating table to begin a site on their own. By the time the hospital heard of these plans and made an offer, agreements had been signed, and it was too late for them to acquire controlling interest in the unit.

Physicians carried out a clandestine campaign to acquire a scanner without hospital involvement when relations between doctors and managers at the hospital were severely strained prior to any discussions on MRI. Often, physician-investor groups held secret meetings and contracted with intermediaries to speed up the siting process. Although hospitals were invariably alerted to the plans before the unit became operational, administrators could not wrestle significant control from the "offending" doctors, often because prior animosities were so acute. The unit was installed while embittered managers talked of setting up their own competing unit in the near future.

The extreme version of this scenario might be termed the *orphan MRI*, where a unit was installed and operated with no hospital involvement whatsoever. We did not come across this situation in the case studies. Nevertheless, our survey data indicate that approximately 50% of all MRI units were installed with no hospital investment whatsoever, suggesting that orphan MRIs may have been a part of the early diffusion process.

Environmental Factors Affecting Diffusion

While the bargaining scenarios were similar in all four markets we visited, the actual pattern of diffusion varied significantly among them. We believe that these differences can be explained, at least in part, by the nature of the competitive market in each community and the relative power of hospitals and physicians in these markets. Population and geography, the insurance market, the regulatory climate, physician density, and the relative economic prosperity in the cities we visited all played a role in how MRI diffused over time.

Population and the economic climate in the metropolitan areas we visited shaped hospital and physician expectations regarding the types of services they could render in the area. Sunnydale and Belle City are medium-sized cities (300,000–500,000), not particularly prosperous, and not expanding as rapidly as other cities in the sunbelt. Prairie City and Metropolis, in contrast, each have populations exceeding 1 million people and large white-collar work forces. No hospital in Sunnydale or Belle City, including the university hospital and the major private tertiary care center, expressed concern with being on the cutting edge of technology. There was, however, intense competition for primary care services among those (few) patients with generous third-party insurance. In contrast, several hospitals in Prairie City and Metropolis considered themselves to be major technology centers. Competition among hospitals in these cities for severely ill patients was much more intense, particularly for those patients with traditional, cost-based, fee-for-service insurance coverage. Finally, the spirit of cooperation among hospitals for sharing services was greater in the prosperous regions since competition for a (relatively) small proportion of individuals with private health insurance was less of an issue in these areas.

The characteristics of the insurance market in each city played a role in hospitals' ability (although not necessarily desire) to acquire MRI. Market penetration by prepaid health plans (HMOs) ranged from less than 10% in Belle City to over 35% of insured patients in Sunnydale. No one we spoke with was happy with the HMOs (although the HMO market share in Belle City was so small that prepaid health plans were hardly an issue). With regards to MRI, HMOs created a very uncomfortable dilemma for hospitals. The majority of managers in all the cities we visited were concerned with attracting HMO patients (where MRI may be an asset), yet once the HMO contracts were signed, services per HMO patient had to be reduced (MRI now became a liability). This problem was compounded in cities where HMOs dominated the market (e.g., Sunnydale), and thus were able to arrange discounted payment contracts with hospitals. HMOs also created (or added to) tensions in hospitals between managers, who sought to reduce services per patient (several administrators in Sunnydale complained that their doctors were "out of control" with regards to ordering tests), and physicians, who cared primarily about adhering to medically-established standards of patient care.

The regulatory climate varied substantially in the cities we visited. At one end of the spectrum was Sunnydale, a city in a state that eliminated its CON laws and state planning agency in 1983, thereby removing all direct government hindrances to acquiring new, expensive medical devices. The other cities had standing CON statutes and state planning agencies that initially allowed only a certain number of certificates for hospital-based MRI units in the area. (None of the states we visited subjected nonhospital outpatient care facilities to CON review.) The permits were always initially given to the largest hospitals in the city. Still, in every case, MRI demand quickly outstripped supply, and hospitals and doctors responded to eliminate the gap. In Prairie City, where ties between hospital leaders and government were close, hospital administrators worked to speed up the CON process and to get additional sites approved, with general success. In Metropolis, hospitals and doctors generally bypassed the process entirely, setting up units off hospital grounds, often applying for CON approval only after the MRI unit had been operating for some time. CON applications were made in these instances, according to administrators and physicians, because it was felt that CON approval conferred "legitimacy" upon the MRI unit—at least in the minds of health professionals who had become accustomed to the CON process—and therefore might make doctors less reluctant to send patients to the MRI facility. In Metropolis, 12 units sprung up during a time when the local Health Systems Agency decided only 6 were needed. All of the CON-approved units were located at major teaching hospitals, while over three-fourths of the nonapproved units were located within walking distance of community hospitals.

Finally, the density of physicians in the area had some effect on ownership and siting of MRI in conflicting ways. On the one hand, hospitals in physician-dense areas were less susceptible to doctors' pressures to acquire units compared to hospitals in other areas. Physicians had little bargaining power in terms of taking their business elsewhere since more doctors could easily be found to fill the void. On the other hand, having a large pool of doctors willing to lend capital for setting up an MRI center made physician-entrepreneurs less dependent on hospitals for setting up MRI units. The result of these forces and the bargaining processes outlined above meant that units in physician-dense areas were more likely to be located outside of hospitals and to have at least partial physician investment. The only city with a relatively low supply of doctors, Prairie City, had few joint ventures and only one unit (a mobile MRI) that was not directly attached to a hospital facility.

CONCLUSIONS AND ISSUES FOR THE FUTURE OF MRI

The manner in which MRI had diffused as of the end of 1986 provides insights into how hospitals have responded to an increasingly uncertain and risky health care environment. Interestingly, the effects of external change on the technology investment decision-making process in hospitals have not led to noticeable changes in the aggregate rate of technology diffusion. MRI is diffusing relatively rapidly. What has changed dramatically, however, is the pattern of diffusion. Hospitals are less willing to bear the entire financial risk associated with MRI and are engaging in a variety of risk-sharing arrangements with other interested parties. In addition, a large number of new entities have been created to own and operate the technology independent of the hospital. How viable these entities will prove to be over the long term is unclear, but they are in competition with hospitals and represent another source of possible erosion in the hospital's revenue base. Thus, the decision process at the hospital level is likely to be influenced by beliefs about competitors' strategies more intensively than ever before, making this process vulnerable to all of the distortions that accompany decisions made under conditions of high uncertainty and intense competition. The field interviews we conducted highlight three important findings that were not evident from the other parts of the study. First, the initial diffusion of scanners was slow, largely due to the high cost of installing and operating units, uncertainties regarding insurer reimbursement for scans, and MRI's unclear clinical advantages over computerized tomography. The earliest MRI procurement was largely traditional (i.e., through hospital purchase), signalling that many physicians shared managers' uncertainties regarding the future of MRI.

As the reimbursement climate cleared and clinical niches for MRI became apparent, physicians (radiologists in particular) grew eager to acquire MRI. The financing options devised by physicians (with and without hospitals), including joint ventures, leasing from intermediaries, and self-financing from physician-dominated funding pools, were a response to their belief that hospitals were unable to acquire units because of regulatory, financial, or space restrictions. These alternatives also demonstrate that physicians have been willing to go to lengths of risk sharing not seen with previous technologies (CT, in particular) to get access to this technology. Perhaps physicians also recognized (as managers may not) the financial and clinical opportunities provided by MRI. For example, physicians may appreciate that as yet unrealized potential applications of MRI (for example, in cardiac imaging) may completely change this technology's future, changing it from a CT-clone to a safer, more accurate, and possibly less-expensive replacement for a host of invasive diagnostic procedures.

Second, MRI demonstrates the dilemma hospital administrators are feeling in balancing the desire to acquire new technologies with the control, legal, and ethical ramifications involved in bringing physicians into the purchasing process. As Medicare ratchets-down DRG payments in the future and if payments for capital and equipment are folded in to PPS, these tensions may become even more acute.

Finally, the variety of decision-process scenarios outlined here suggests that the new environment is significantly affecting doctor-hospital relationships and dynamics. PPS is only one of myriad changes facing the health care enterprise in the 1980s. Traditional forms of negotiation and ownership seem to be breaking down, in part, due to PPS. The case of MRI may thus portend a new era in the diffusion of sophisticated, high-cost medical technological devices—one where hospitals, physicians, and corporate health care enterprises are willing to share the risks (and benefits) of bringing new medical technology to patients, and where the hospital may become less dominant as the locus of high technology.

NOTE

1. The study defines freestanding imaging organizations (FIO) as diagnostic centers located off hospital grounds. These centers are often owned in part by a hospital. FIOs usually offer a range of diagnostic imaging services, including (for example) MRI, CT scanning, and ultrasound.

PART III
TECHNOLOGY AND THE CHANGING ENVIRONMENT

13

The Legal and Economic Realities for Health Technology in the United States

Paul C. Rettig

It is often stated that the United States has the best medical care in the world. This statement usually refers to the unprecedented access, for most patients, to sophisticated technological intervention that has characterized U.S. medicine for much of the 20th century. The result has been a saving of lives, relief of pain, and improvement in the quality of life that has occurred on a scale previously unknown in the world of medicine.

To a great extent, the unique U.S. system of fee-for-service payment for medical care has been responsible for this widespread access to sophisticated technology. The average patient has been largely shielded from the high cost of technological intervention by a system whereby private insurers have reimbursed providers retrospectively, with little thought to cost efficiency. Thus new technologies could be brought into the marketplace with little concern about cost.

This situation has changed drastically. Since the 1970s the skyrocketing cost of health care has led to a growing emphasis on cost efficiency. As this book shows, this new perspective has had dramatic effects on the nature and utilization of medical technology. There is financial incentive for only those technologies that can enhance a hospital's financial position under Medicare's Prospective Payment System (PPS). Not only the cost of care but also the quality of care may be affected in coming years. If the environment is hostile to the development and implementation of new technology, patients may have to do without valuable treatments that might otherwise have been developed.

Before an entrepreneur or a company can work to implement new ideas for medical technology, the eventual profitability of the technology must be considered. This is a long-term consideration; the profit will not be realized in the short term. The time, investment, and opportunity costs involved in developing a new technology must be weighed against its money-making potential over time. Two factors are especially important: the length of time it will take to get the new technology to market, and the price the technology will command.

These factors depend upon several variables. A new technology must first be submitted to the complex regulatory mechanisms of the Food and Drug Administration (FDA), which approves a new technology before it can enter the market. This review can often take years. After a technology is approved, it must then be classified for Medicare payment under PPS by the Health Care Financing Administration (HCFA), which decides upon an appropriate diagnosis-related group (DRG) in which to put the technology, and also decides upon an appropriate payment level. This process presents several significant obstacles to the implementation of new technology: aside from the additional time required for HCFA's decision-making process, the eventual payment rates or payment arrangements for some technologies might prove inadequate.

In addition to the time spent in arriving at these regulatory decisions, the element of uncertainty involved can be daunting. Will the FDA and Medicare approvals take one year or six? Will payment arrangements make any particular product financially viable or not? Not knowing, and thus being forced to rely on educated guesses, is part of the reality of introducing new technology into the post-PPS health care marketplace.

FDA APPROVALS OF NEW PRODUCTS

Under the 1976 Medical Device amendments to the Food, Drug, and Cosmetic Act, medical devices are subject to regulation by the Food and Drug Administration. Devices that incorporate significant new technologies can normally be marketed only after they receive a premarket approval (PMA) from the FDA.

Depending upon the data provided by the developer of the new technology and upon its similarity to other already existing technologies, this process can be lengthy. It is a difficult, complex process, often hindered by bureaucratic delay as well as delays resulting from the usual technological and scientific complications that typically arise in research of this type. One 1985 study of selected new technologies showed that FDA review times for these technologies averaged over five years (Bucci, Reiss & Hall, 1985). The selected technologies studied included devices such as the implantable pump, cochlear implant, artificial knee, artificial hip, lithotriptor, and heart valve. For all new technologies that require premarket approval—not just selected devices—the average review time is shorter, but still well over a year. FDA reports 395 days as the average review time for final premarket approvals during fiscal year 1986 (Food and Drug Administration, 1986). The medical device industry is concerned about delays in product approvals and has lobbied Congress to urge additional funds and staffing for FDA in hope of speeding up FDA product reviews.

Premarket approval requires an application to the FDA that includes voluminous and complex information. The objective is to provide enough information to enable the FDA to determine that the medical device is "safe and effective." Normally this will include information on clinical trials conducted on patients. The process is time consuming and resource consuming both for the manufacturer and for the FDA. An alternative route to legal marketing of a product may occur if the product is substantially equivalent to a product that was on the market before 1976. This is a kind of grandfather clause in the 1976 law that subjects a device to the same level of regulatory review as the pre–1976 device to which it is substantially equivalent. In practice, the great majority, perhaps 98%, of new products get to market this way. Even pacemakers, which might be thought to be in a class of products most risky and therefore most needing premarket approval, do not require it, because the pre–1976 device had not been subject to it. Manufacturers are required, however, to submit significant information to the FDA about their products when claiming substantial equivalence; in practice, this has often included the submission of clinical data.

Congressional discontent with this regulatory process is reflected in the title of a 1983 report by the Subcommittee on Oversight and Investigations of the House Committee on Energy and Commerce: "Medical Device Regulation: The FDA's Neglected Child," and in a number of oversight and legislative hearings held by that subcommittee and the Committee's Subcommittee on Health and the Environment.

In July 1988, the House Committee on Energy and Commerce ordered report H.R. 4640, the "Medical Device Improvement Act of 1988," designed to respond to congressional concerns that the regulatory FDA process needed revision both on the grounds that some unsafe products might be finding their way to market and on the grounds that some changes in regulatory priorities and FDA staff resource allocations may be needed.

In general, the bill attempts to assure that products are more appropriately classified and reclassified by the FDA in terms of the risks inherent in their use, with the end result that regulatory emphasis in product approval will be placed on the most risky devices and that the way to market for the others will be eased. An important feature of the bill, a separate new requirement that health care providers report directly to the FDA cases in which a medical device may have caused or contributed to the death of a patient, is designed to improve the ability to catch unsafe products that might get to market as a result of eased approval procedures.

Considerable negotiation and discussion between House committee personnel and manufacturers' representatives preceded committee approval of this legislation. Manufacturers are eager to get products to market but are fully amenable to regulation that requires not only themselves but also their competitors to demonstrate that their products are safe and effective.

Consumers are not well-represented in this highly technical area. On occasion, groups such as the Health Research Group, originating with Ralph Nader, attempt to represent them. The FDA has the responsibility of assuring the safety of medical devices but is interested also in administrative feasibility and always faces staff resource limitations in carrying out its product approval responsibilities. For the moment, these interests seem to have been accommodated sufficiently to prevent any party from becoming so distressed as to mount a serious effort to defeat the legislation.

MEDICARE COVERAGE

FDA approval means that a product can be legally marketed. In some cases, however, Medicare and other third-party payers may be unprepared for new technology and may not pay for it until it is better understood. A significant new technology, especially if it is costly or if it is expected to be widely used, will come to the special attention of staff at the Health Care Financing Administration (HCFA). There, the question of whether the technology should be covered by Medicare will be examined. If the HCFA staff cannot resolve the question, a special physician review panel at HCFA will be asked for advice. In turn, that panel may request an assessment by the Public Health Service Office of Health Technology Assessment (OHTA).

As a practical matter, the great majority of questions that arise about coverage of technologies are handled at the staff level without referral to the physician panel. In many cases the technology is clearly excluded by existing Medicare law, or a previous coverage decision is clearly applicable. In other cases, the technology is similar enough that the staff feels able to make a decision based on analogy to the decision already made. According to HCFA staff, perhaps 80% of the first inquiries can be handled at the staff level. A medical device manufacturer may inquire, for example, about a product in development, whether it will be covered, and what data HCFA will need to make a coverage determination. Later, when the manufacturer actually requests a coverage determination, the issue may need to go to the physician panel. Perhaps two or three out of four do go to the panel.

In deciding whether a coverage issue merits a national policy decision, criteria such as the following are considered: whether conflicting interpretations are being made by different Medicare carriers, whether there are public health concerns relating to safety of the technology, whether there is likely to be rapid diffusion of the technology, whether coverage presents a financial risk to the Medicare program, and to what degree the technology presents a risk of program abuse.

The physician panel is informally constituted at present, but includes physicians not only from HCFA but also physician representation from the Public Health Service. It meets at fairly regular intervals: every six to eight weeks in the past, somewhat less frequently recently. The physician panel is sometimes able to make a definitive decision, but often the decision is whether the issue should go to OHTA for a full assessment. On occasion, data and advice are requested from OHTA on the question of whether a full assessment would be appropriate. Relatively few coverage issues are sent to OHTA for full assessment, usually approximately 12 to 18 per year.

Like the review by FDA, this Medicare coverage review can take time. In some cases the delay will be long. In the decade ending in 1985, most decisions were made in less than three years. Fortunately, the review time has been declining. From 1983 to 1985, the average was about a year and a half. There is still considerable variation: MRI took about three and a half years. The implantable automatic defibrillator took less than one year.

Regulatory lag is not the only problem with Medicare coverage reviews. It is not clear what criteria are used in making the coverage decision. Medicare law uses the vague phrase *reasonable and necessary*. The concept of *safe and effective* is also used, but how this differs from FDA determination criteria for safety and effectiveness is not clear. Cost effectiveness is a criterion that is mentioned in laws relating to OHTA's review of technologies, but the Medicare law itself does not specify cost effectiveness as a criterion that may be used.

Another problem with this decision-making process is its isolation from public opinion and input. There are no formal opportunities for public contribution to the process. There is evidence, however, of growing official awareness of this problem. The Department of Health and Human Services itself has been studying the strengths and weaknesses of the coverage process, and the Administrative Conference of the United States has urged more openness and regularity in Medicare coverage decision-making.

Medicare has long excluded "experimental" items from coverage. This concept, at times, appears to have been misapplied. In 1982, a successful balloon catheter coronary angioplasty (PTCA) procedure was denied coverage as an "experimental" procedure, although the type of catheter used had already been approved by the FDA as safe and effective. In a settlement of the ensuing case, the Department of Health and Human Services agreed (in addition to payment of the patient's expenses) that HCFA would publish in the Federal Register a description of the process it uses to make Medicare coverage decisions, and a description of the criteria it uses. HCFA has published a description of the process and has asked for public comment on both the process and the coverage criteria.

As of August 1988, HCFA had in the final stages of internal review a notice of proposed rulemaking (NPRM) containing detailed descriptions of the Medicare coverage process with HCFA. It was reported to include considerable detail on the process and the steps involved in making a coverage determination, including the criteria to be used in selecting issues for which a national policy appears to be needed, and criteria to be used in deciding the coverage issue itself. The proposed rule reportedly will include "cost effectiveness" as a criterion that may be used, will describe several methodologies for measuring cost effectiveness, and will request public comment on the cost-effectiveness issue and the methodologies. This proposed rule was not expected to address in any detail the process and criteria used by OHTA in making Medicare coverage recommendations, but OHTA in turn was reported to be revising its own procedures and criteria and preparing to publish descriptions of them. These developments give hope of changes that will smooth the path for Medicare coverage of technologies.

A final problem with Medicare coverage is an antiquated benefit definition. Medical technology has made the safe performance of complex care outside the institutional setting possible. Under Medicare, a procedure that moves from an inpatient to an ambulatory care setting will become eligible for coverage under Part B rather than Part A. Part B, however, contains a list of services covered; if a service is not listed, it will not be covered. With few exceptions, this listing, which was developed in 1965, is still law. Thus electronic bone growth stimulators are covered, but not necessarily the intensive technical services performed by the manufacturer for each patient using the device. Coverage of these services depends upon sympathetic bureaucratic interpretation of the Part B stipulations. Until recently, home antibiotic infusion therapy was not covered at all, although it is much less expensive than the same procedure done in-hospital. Only with the passage of P.L. 100–360 on July 1, 1988, was Medicare law changed to cover home IV drug therapy.

MEDICARE PAYMENT

Technology development is moving in the direction of emphasizing those technologies that will reduce costs. Professional concern for quality may motivate providers not to choose the ''cost-saving'' technology in every instance, but DRG restrictions have made it essential to be especially vigilant of the costs and benefits of every procedure, service, and facility offered. Technologies that will reduce length of stay, reduce utilization of ancillary services, and lower the price of materials and supplies are expected to be emphasized in the current cost-conscious atmosphere.

Also important will be technologies that will facilitate a reduction in staffing levels and an increase in admissions, along with an increasing specialization in services. Technologies that do not carry with them an implicit guarantee of cost saving may not be in high demand. Medical supply firms seem not to have made major changes in research and development, but they are looking earlier at marketability in this cost-sensitive environment (Lewin & Associates, Inc., 1987).

Whether these trends will truly result in lowering of costs remains to be seen. It is possible that competition may take the form of competition for real or perceived quality, even if this means investing in and utilizing technology that is not the most cost saving available. Hospitals are currently being criticized for increasing their costs more rapidly than PPS payments are increasing, even as their operating margins are shrinking drastically. Nonetheless, the emphasis on cost saving under PPS makes it essential that a new technology be seen as cost effective as well as high-quality and efficient.

Thus the final decision about payment for individual technologies is not the only important consideration. At least as important for the continued development of new technologies is the *expectation* of fair and adequate payment. This is why it is important to provide the greatest possible assurance that beneficial medical technologies will be adequately reimbursed. The Prospective Payment Assessment Commission (ProPAC) plays an important role in providing this assurance. One of ProPAC's specific charges under Medicare law is to advise on technological advances and the issue of medical technology that increases cost but also improves quality.

A bill introduced by Senator Durenberger (R., Minn.) also addresses this issue. To encourage continued innovation, the bill provides a temporary additional payment for technologies or procedures adopted by a hospital where use of the technology raises costs for a particular DRG significantly beyond Medicare's DRG payment (U.S. Congress, Senate, 1987).

RESPONSE TO THE PAYMENT AND MARKET ENVIRONMENT

The technology industry continues to grow. Shipments of medical and surgical instruments and supplies are expected to reach $21.1 billion in 1987—an 8.5% real growth increase over 1986. The Commerce Department expects that the long-term prospects for continued growth in the industry will be very dependent upon a high degree of innovation. A survey of device and diagnostic manufacturers showed that they invested an average of 7.5% of 1985 sales on research and development. This is more than twice the rate for the manufacturing sector as a whole.[1] R&D spending was a significant strategy in responding to market changes caused by the start of Medicare's Prospective Payment System (PPS).

Sixty percent of the companies in the survey reported that PPS did not change their basic research and development strategy. But 40% did change their strategy in the first year after PPS, and these companies tended to focus on developing cost-effective products with short-term payoffs.

One more economic reality affecting the development of medical technology should be mentioned here: skyrocketing product liability insurance premiums and high damage awards. According to a recent survey, several medical technology companies have abandoned entire product lines rather than face the potential liability associated with these medical products. Among the products dropped were radiation therapy devices, defibrillators, infant ventilators, pacemakers, contraceptive devices, fracture fixation devices, a drill used during brain surgery, and a pump used in bypass surgery. Several companies also reported that they would not pursue the development of certain products because of product liability concerns.

Discussed less often, but essential to this issue, is long-term liability of new technology. Insurance against claims that might come along many years after the procedure is one of the most important facets in the raising of product liability costs. As more technologies are developed that will allow patients who would otherwise have died to survive for longer periods of time, long-term liability will become an increasingly important issue, needing extensive further research and careful consideration on the part of technology developers.

CONCLUSION

Developing new medical technology and bringing it to market are expensive propositions. In considering whether to develop a product, costs of complying with regulation and dealing with regulatory lag will be important, regardless of how desirable and necessary this regulation may be to assure product safety and effectiveness. The further delay, outlined in this chapter, in getting Medicare and other payers to recognize and provide coverage for new technologies is a relatively recent development affecting this decision. In the new economic environment under PPS and managed health care, additional challenges face those who attempt to decide upon research and development of medical technology.

Little evidence exists thus far that technological innovation has suffered under PPS. Changes may have occurred in the emphasis of research and development toward products that will promise short-term savings to health care providers. There is little empirical evidence, however, that technologies that will increase costs have suffered.

It is currently unclear what the future may hold. The early years of PPS have not put undue pressure upon hospitals. This may change, however, and hospital behavior under PPS, struggling with DRGs, may change in ways adverse to new medical technology. Medicare Part B premiums will rise by nearly 40% in the coming year. This drastic increase will most likely portend major new cost-cutting efforts under Medicare Part B.

Public and private payers can also be expected to examine technology more closely with respect to its value in improving health outcomes. There will be greater efforts to define and measure quality of care and to use new techniques to examine the value of individual medical technologies. Greater efforts to determine whether a technology is a real improvement over previous technologies can be expected; also increasingly examined will be whether the improvement is worth the increased cost. Greater attention will be paid to the usefulness and appropriateness of technologies in specific situations; some technologies may be authorized by some payers for selective coverage limited to specific situations.

As frustration over apparently inexorable increases in health care cost grow, we can expect more vocal condemnations of medical technology as well as further attempts to limit and control it directly. Further regulatory pressures may lead to diminished competitive power in the international market. Financial and regulatory constraints may hinder U.S. suppliers and developers of technology in getting their products to foreign markets, giving an advantage to competitors in other countries with less-restrictive regulatory pressures. Since investment money can be used for a variety of purposes, there is a danger that the difficulties presented by some of the regulatory problems outlined in this chapter could eventually cause investors to steer their money in different directions. A potentially serious slowdown in research and development of new medical technologies could result.

Legal and economic problems such as these facing health technology development are real, and must be addressed. Thus far, however, technology development seems not to have been seriously compromised. In the current climate of cost consciousness and increased competition and volatility, this could change. The situation bears watching, and further research will be needed to identify and predict these trends.

NOTE

1. Health Industry Manufacturers' Association member survey (internal organizational memorandum).

14

Implications of Recent Medicare
Changes upon Hospital Technology

David G. Whiteis and Ross M. Mullner

With the passage of Medicare's Prospective Payment System (PPS) in 1983, the financial incentives facing the nation's hospitals changed dramatically. In general, the new incentives encouraged hospitals to:

1. reduce the cost of treating patients over the course of their hospital stay;

2. increase the number of admissions, especially for particular groups of patients; and

3. develop new sources of revenue not subject to payment restrictions. (Office of Technology Assessment, 1985)

Hospitals have pursued various specific strategies in dealing with the new system. Among these are decreasing the cost of admission (through reductions in length of stay and reduction in ancillary services, staffing levels, and supply prices); increasing admissions, particularly for those patients with profitable diagnosis-related groups (DRGs); increasing readmissions and interhospital transfers; increasing discharges to nursing homes; integrating hospital services with noninstitutional services such as nursing homes and home health care agencies; increasing specialization of services; "upcoding" diagnoses and procedures reported for payment purposes; and increasing hospital diversification into provision of unregulated health services (Office of Technology Assessment, 1985).

After implementation of PPS, hospitals' net patient-revenue margins (surpluses derived from the treatment of patients) rose. Since 1985, however, revenue margins have declined precipitously. For example, in 1985 and 1986, revenue margins for the nation's community hospitals decreased from 1.5% to 0.7% and for the year ending September 1987 they dropped from 0.6% to 0.2%. In 1986, more than half of all community hospitals actually lost money on patient care (American Hospital Association, 1988).

As margins continue to fall, there is growing concern that hospitals' ability to channel resources into essential community services, patient care, and new medical technology may be affected. Hospitals may be unable to purchase new technology because of lack of funds. Further, new technology that fails to fit the dollar limit that Medicare or other third-party payers prescribe for the course of treatment may not be purchased. Technological development may be more limited than in the past, with an emphasis on cost-cutting technologies that will quickly find their way into use (Rubin et al., 1988).

According to a recent report:

Reimbursement affects hospitals' ability to purchase new technology. Many systems encourage the purchase of only cost-saving technology. Consequently, our nation's medical research and development efforts may be limited, thereby slowing the introduction of new diagnostic and treatment techniques.

When hospital payment was based upon the actual costs of the care provided and when the capital costs associated with equipment expenditures were reimbursed in full, new technology was adopted relatively quickly. There are early indications that this might not occur under new payment systems.

Under the Medicare Prospective Payment System, for example, if a technology was in place in 1981 when the system was developed, the costs for use of that technology were included in the DRG payment amount. For technology becoming available after that time, the costs are not included. Unless Medicare explicitly adopts the new technology and incorporates it into the payment system, hospitals will not be reimbursed for its use. Hospitals, therefore, have an incentive to adopt a new technology only if it reduces the costs of providing services, thereby allowing them to benefit from the cost savings. Any technology that adds to the costs of patient care could mean potential financial losses for the hospital. (Rubin et al., 1988)

The objective of this chapter is twofold. First, it will discuss the impact of PPS upon the development, diffusion, and type of medical technology hospitals are likely to adopt in the future. Second, it will discuss some of the problems and difficulties of incorporating new technology into PPS. Three new technologies will be discussed: lithotripsy, magnetic resonance imaging, and cochlear implants. Also discussed will be the actual decision-making process devised by the Prospective Payment Assessment Commission (ProPAC) to fit new technologies into the PPS system. It is hoped that by comparing this formalized process with the actual case studies, the reader will gain an understanding of both the strengths and weaknesses of the process.

POTENTIAL IMPACTS

Although it is very difficult to measure the impact of PPS for a number of reasons (i.e., the complexity of the interactions among the incentives under PPS and the constraints faced by hospitals and other providers), the Office of Technology Assessment (OTA) has identified a number of likely changes in hospital behavior. Table 14.1 summarizes the relationship between the predicted changes in hospital behavior and the potential impacts upon technological change and clinical research.

The primary initial assumption behind PPS was that a significant amount of unnecessary or inefficient care had been delivered in hospitals prior to its inception. Thus cost containment could be achieved by trimming the fat from the health care delivery system while retaining those services, facilities, and procedures that were truly necessary for good care. Resources could be conserved, and procedures of little benefit to patients would be eliminated.

In practice, the ability of hospitals to respond to incentives put in place under PPS depends largely upon the amount of economic pressure they must endure in an increasingly competitive and volatile health care marketplace. This is especially true for not-for-profit hospitals, which represent the vast majority of hospitals in the United States (American Hospital Association, 1987). When weighing options for strategic or technological responses to PPS, hospitals must increasingly consider the potential for revenue gains, the cost of implementation, whether the strategy or technology fits the objectives of management and medical staff, and the potential impact on patient care (Office of Technology Assessment, 1985).

PPS is structured on a per-case basis, with DRG categories defining the payment level for these cases. Most of the potential impacts of PPS are due to its per-case nature and to the DRG classification system. The profitability of an individual patient is largely defined before that patient is treated. Former strategies such as cost shifting, whereby patients needing relatively inexpensive treatment would be charged somewhat higher to help offset the cost of treating expensive patients, become difficult or impossible under PPS.

Thus a new array of strategies has become necessary for hospitals to achieve the goal of per-case cost reductions. Summarizing recent studies and projections of future hospital behavior, OTA (1985) has identified several likely hospital tactics to reduce per-admission costs. These include:

1. reduction of lengths of stay;
2. reduction of the use of ancillary services;
3. reduction of staffing levels and of the personnel/patient ratio, and also reducing rates of employee fringe benefits and wages;
4. offering traditional inpatient technologies and services on an outpatient basis;
5. increasing the development of low-cost technologies, and purchasing supplies and equipment with an increased emphasis on frugality;

Table 14.1
Summary of Potential PPS Impacts on Technological Change and Clinical Research

Predicted Changes in Hospital Behavior	Potential Impacts
Length of Stay (down)	May increase research on and adoption and use of technologies that lower cost by lowering length of stay; may decrease development and diffusion of those that raise length of stay.
Ancillary Services (down)	May increase development and diffusion of technologies that permit fewer or less frequent ancillary services; may decrease development and diffusion of those that require more.
Prices of Materials and Supplies (down)	May decrease research and development by private industry.
Use of Less-Expensive Materials and Supplies (up)	May increase development and diffusion of supply technologies (such as wound dressing) that lower costs; may decrease development and diffusion of those that raise them.
Staffing Levels (down)	May increase research on and adoption and use of technologies that are less labor-intensive; may decrease development and diffusion of those that are more labor-intensive.
Admissions (up)	May increase clinical research and technology adoption and use in profitable DRG's; may decrease them in unprofitable ones.

Readmissions (up)	No effect.
Transfers (up)	No effect.
Discharges to Nursing Homes (up)	May encourage more clinical research in nursing home settings.
Discharges to Home Health Care (up)	May encourage more clinical research in home settings; may increase development and diffusion of technologies that can be used at home.
Vertical Integration of Services (up)	May increase diffusion of traditional inpatient technologies into outpatient and home settings.
Specialization of Services (up)	May encourage research on and adoption of technologies in hospital's area of specialization in order to enhance hospital's reputation.
Upcoding (up)	May encourage adoption and use of technologies that permit patient to be classified into a higher-paying DRG (when resulting additional reimbursement is greater than additional cost).

Source: Office of Technology Assessment, 1985

189

6. reduction of activities such as continuing education and clinical research by moving these activities into nonhospital settings such as nursing homes and home care.

While lowering the per-case cost of care, hospitals are also motivated to increase those admissions that will be profitable under DRG payment restrictions. Specifically, incentives are in place to encourage such strategies as:

1. attracting relatively healthy patients through marketing and the offering of services these patients will use;
2. treating some patients on an inpatient basis who would otherwise be considered ambulatory patients;
3. encouraging multiple admissions for a single patient rather than one prolonged hospital stay;
4. decreasing staffing levels in expensive specialties while increasing them in areas that are more cost effective; and
5. increasing referrals of unprofitable patients to other institutions, especially public hospitals. (Office of Technology Assessment, 1985)

The final area in which hospitals will be encouraged to implement cost-saving strategies involves expansion into services that will be more profitable and less constrained under PPS. Especially significant is ambulatory care, which continues to be reimbursed under Medicare on a cost basis.

A number of factors contribute to the growth of outpatient care in the post-PPS era. Technological advancement has greatly increased the number of surgical procedures that can be performed on an outpatient basis (Henderson, 1987); peer review organizations (PROs) are under contractual arrangements with the Health Care Financing Administration (HCFA) to review whether inpatient admissions are appropriate and necessary; and the cost to physicians of performing surgical procedures on an outpatient basis is considerably less. These factors are predicted to lead to a rapid growth of ambulatory surgery in the future.

It is important to note that some of the incentives under PPS may be contradictory. While ambulatory procedures are favored over expensive inpatient care as a way of lowering per-case cost, the need to increase admissions may yet spur hospitals to treat on an inpatient basis some patients who would otherwise receive ambulatory care (Enthoven & Noll, 1984). In addition, surgical procedures (except for those classified as experimental) are itemized individually under PPS, as contrasted to the prepayment model in private HMOs, where the annual or monthly charge covers all medical care, including surgery (Bunker & Schaffarzick, 1986). An incentive thus remains in place to perform surgery and in some cases to inflate DRG payment to a level close to that of pre-DRG cost-based reimbursement (Bunker & Schaffarzick, 1986).

Moreover, while investment in expensive new technology is theoretically discouraged, hospitals will also face stiff competition for physicians and patients and thus be under continued pressure to invest in expensive technological equipment to attract doctors (Steinberg & Cohen, 1984). This tension between the need to cut cost and the need to fill beds is a significant component of the pressure on providers under PPS.

To summarize, three basic strategies are predicted to dominate hospital behavior under PPS: lowering per-case cost; increasing the number of profitable admissions while de-emphasizing those that will be unprofitable; and expanding into services and technologies that are either well-paid under PPS or not constrained by PPS restrictions. The twin incentives to reduce length of stay and increase admissions create a somewhat contradictory situation for hospitals and planners attempting to devise profitable strategies under PPS. The emphasis will increasingly be on low-cost, high-return technologies that will attract patients to the hospital, allow them to be diagnosed in such a way that they will fit into well-paid DRGs, and facilitate their early discharge. Patients needing further care will increasingly be discharged into a home care setting or nursing homes.

More specifically, research and development of health care technology is likely to become increasingly focused in those areas that will be most profitable. Technologies that will reduce length of stay, be less labor intensive, and utilized in profitable DRG categories will likely become a high priority in the post-PPS era.

Hospitals may be encouraged to invest in technologies that will allow a patient to be classified in as high paying a DRG as possible. It has been suggested that this may contradict the stated intention of PPS to discourage unnecessary intervention and care; especially significant in this regard is the fact that nonexperimental surgical procedures are itemized individually under PPS. This allows inflation and "DRG creep" to interfere with the cost-cutting mechanism and may provide an incentive for unnecessary surgical intervention as well.

Incentives to discharge patients into home care programs or nursing homes may encourage a greater emphasis on clinical research resulting in the proliferation of new technologies and treatments designed to be administered in these settings. Conversely, expensive ancillary services are expected to decrease under PPS, leading to a concomitant slowdown in the development of technologies that require such services and the proliferation of technologies that restrict their number or frequency.

It is apparent that the implementation of PPS has significant implications for the nature of health care technology. As research and scientific breakthroughs introduce new diagnostic and treatment technologies, health care providers must keep up with these advances while remaining mindful of the restrictions inherent in PPS. The tension between keeping pace with new technological developments while maintaining cost effectiveness will result in serious challenges for hospitals and other health care providers.

The following section will illustrate some of these difficulties by examining three technologies—extracorporeal shock wave lithotripsy (ESWL), magnetic resonance imaging (MRI), and cochlear implants—in light of federal attempts to classify them into appropriate DRGs.

INCORPORATING NEW TECHNOLOGY UNDER PPS: PROBLEMS AND DIFFICULTIES

The decision-making process involved in the adoption of new technology under the PPS system is complex and difficult. The Prospective Payment Assessment Commission (ProPAC) is the federal body charged with the responsibility of recommending to HCFA the appropriate classification, under PPS, for a new technology or procedure.

To fit diseases and medical procedures into DRGs, a coding system known as ICD–9–CM (International Classification of Diseases, 9th Clinical Modification), or simply ICD–9, was adapted by HCFA from the field of epidemiology. It was initially developed by scientists to study the relative frequency of different diseases (Wild, 1987). ICD–9–CM is comprised of both a comprehensive list of diseases with corresponding codes and a list of procedure codes. The World Health Organization (WHO) maintains and updates the codes (Office of Technology Assessment, 1985).

DRG assignment depends upon both disease and procedure codes. A patient is put in a major diagnostic category by the disease code, indicating which of several DRGs may be appropriate. A code for a principal procedure, or its absence, is then used to define the procedure as either surgical or medical. Based on the specific procedure performed, the age of the patient, and the presence or absence of coexisting diseases and complications, the final choice of a DRG is then made (Office of Technology Assessment, 1985).

The process of fitting a disease or technology into an appropriate DRG involves several decisions: identifying the applicable ICD–9 code (if one exists), categorizing the procedure as surgical or nonsurgical, and deciding whether it is therapeutic or diagnostic. After this classification has been done, an appropriate weight for the DRG to include the cost of this new technology must be calculated. As will be seen in the following case studies, this process can be complex and ambiguous.

Extracorporeal Shock Wave Lithotripsy

Extracorporeal shock wave lithotripsy (ESWL) uses shock waves to break up urinary tract stones without a surgical incision. A related technology, ultrasonic lithotripsy, involves making a small incision in the patient's back and inserting a small endoscopic device known as an ultrasonic lithotriptor to fragment the stone before its removal (Office of Technology Assessment, 1985). ESWL is considered a significant advance over ultrasonic lithotripsy because no incision is required.

Because of its noninvasive nature, ESWL can reduce length of stay for kidney stone patients and can also be offered on an outpatient basis. Thus, even though an extracorporeal shock wave lithotriptor is expensive, it can significantly lower overall hospital costs (Office of Technology Assessment, 1985).

ESWL was not a Medicare-covered service when DRGs were developed in 1983. It was approved by the Food and Drug Administration (FDA) in December 1984, and for Medicare coverage shortly thereafter (Teitelman, 1985). There was no ICD–9 code at the time that recognized this technology. Ultrasonic lithotripsy, however, was already classified under ICD–9 Code No. 59.95. This code is usually used in conjunction with a code for incision to qualify ultrasonic lithotripsy as a minor surgical (percutaneous) procedure, resulting in assignment to a higher-paying surgical DRG (Office of Technology Assessment, 1985).

The initial debate over ESWL centered around whether it should be categorized as surgery. As a procedure involving no surgical incision and usually not performed in an operating room, ESWL was considered by some in HCFA to be an inappropriate candidate for classification as a surgical procedure. On the other hand, others argued, it could be considered an invasive procedure because the shock waves do permeate the skin and disintegrate kidney stones inside the body. Because surgical DRGs are paid for at a higher rate than nonsurgical DRGs, this debate was more than an academic exercise; it had profound implications for health care providers.

The final decision was to categorize ESWL as a medical rather than surgical procedure. The only available ICD–9 category dealing with the disintegration of stones, however, and thus the only one into which ESWL could be fit, was 59.95, the same code used for ultrasonic lithotripsy. When reported without a corresponding code for a surgical incision or other invasive procedure, an ESWL case is classified into one of two DRGs: DRG 323 (Urinary Stones age > 69 and/or C. C. [complications and comorbidities]) or DRG 324 (Urinary Stones age < 70 w/o C. C.). Cases requiring a percutaneous procedure or conventional surgery are grouped into a more expensive DRG: 304 or 305 (ProPAC, 1986).

ProPAC has since reviewed this assignment process. Utilizing cost data from the American Hospital Association (AHA), the American Urological Association (AUA), and seven providers of ESWL, ProPAC found that the per-case cost of ESWL varies widely with the number of ESWL shocks delivered per case. In the ESWL procedure, a disposable electrode is used that costs between $200 and $300; more complex or difficult cases may require the use of more electrodes, although even an average case requires as many as three electrodes per treatment.

Current cost data, ProPAC found, are based on a relatively low volume of cases per hospital. As hospitals begin to use the technology more efficiently, the per-case cost may drop significantly. At the present time, however, the DRG 324 payment rate for ESWL is significantly lower than operating costs, while the DRG 323 payment rate reflects between 80% and 100% of operating costs. If ESWL were reclassified into DRGs 304 and 305, as some analysts have suggested, payments would exceed 200% of operating costs (ProPAC, 1986).

Because of these uncertainties, ProPAC recommended that ESWL be removed from DRG 324 and reassigned entirely to DRG 323. All payments and costs would then be monitored to determine the appropriate payment for operating costs. ProPAC also recommended the identification of a new ICD–9 procedure code for ESWL.

This case illustrates the difficulty involved in fitting medical and surgical procedures into a coding system initially intended for epidemiologic research, and also the increasing obsolescence of traditional concepts such as "surgical," "invasive," and "noninvasive." As the ESWL case illustrates, technology can change and advance more rapidly than policymakers' ability to adapt. Under PPS, which requires classification into preconceived categories in order for a procedure to be covered, the assignment process may become increasingly difficult as technology begins to make old definitions and concepts obsolete.

Magnetic Resonance Imaging

Where ESWL posed a problem because of vagaries in classification and definition, magnetic resonance imaging (MRI) is an example of a technology that can be used in a wide variety of medical procedures, and thus alter costs within many DRGs. It has been estimated that MRI may substitute for up to 30% of other hospital resources (ProPAC, 1986).

MRI uses a scanner to produce images of the internal structure of the head and body; it is a diagnostic rather than a therapeutic technology (ProPAC, 1986). Although in use since the mid–1970s, MRI became covered under Medicare in November 1985. It was therefore not included in data used to develop DRGs and their respective weights in 1983.

MRI is expensive; an average scan in 1986 was estimated to cost approximately $335 (ProPAC, 1986). Hospitals have not rushed to incorporate MRI technology into their mix of facilities and services. The percent of MRI scanners in hospitals is significantly lower than that for computed tomography (CT) scanning (Steinberg, Sisk & Locke, 1985). It was thus felt that Medicare patients had insufficient access to this technology.

In addition, there was a danger that the lack of appropriate PPS payment for MRI scans might lead hospitals to distribute the scanners in outpatient settings, where cost-based reimbursement would result in significantly higher payments. Hospitals could thus circumvent the payment restrictions imposed by PPS. Their patients would then also be responsible under Medicare Part B cost sharing for a 20% copayment. All standard restrictions and liabilities associated with any hospital stay resulting from the procedure would be in place (ProPAC, 1987).

For these reasons, the MRI issue was approached with a sense of urgency. In considering alternatives for the classification and payment for MRI under PPS, several options were considered.

It was suggested that the initial payment mechanism chosen by HCFA during the period when ProPAC was investigating the issue might be the most efficient and equitable. MRI treatment would be covered under Medicare, but the cost of the technology itself would not be covered. Payment would be based upon a standardized amount, the weight of the DRG(s) involved, and adjustments for other expenses such as wages, teaching, and payment for outliers. The standardized amount, as recommended by ProPAC, would include a factor to adjust for cost-increasing and quality-enhancing technologies as they were developed; thus hospitals would already possess some additional funds for utilizing a new technology such as MRI.

According to law, DRG rates must be recalibrated at least once every four years to reflect changes in cost over time; ProPAC recommends an annual recalibration (see Appendix). It would be assumed that as MRI utilization increases, charges for the procedure would begin to appear in the data bases Medicare uses for this recalibration. Thus after a period of time, weights for individual DRGs would include the cost of MRI.

Under this scheme, MRI would be treated the same as other technologies whose use does not necessitate specific changes or adjustments in DRG weights or classifications; as the cost of MRI became apparent in the data, it would be included in the normal periodic recalibration of DRG payment rates.

Unfortunately, this dependence upon an evolutionary process would create a time lag; it might take up to two years for a change in cost brought about by use of MRI to be reflected in the annual recalibration of payment rates. If recalibration were to occur less often, the time lag would be even longer. Because MRI scans are distributed widely through cases falling into numerous DRG categories, there might also be insufficient MRI cases in some DRGs to raise significantly payment levels to reflect the added cost of an MRI scan.

Moreover, this alternative does not take into consideration the fact that MRI is not always used in every appropriate diagnostic situation. If all DRGs in which MRI can be used were eventually reweighted, the new DRG weight (and thus the payment) for any given case would be the same regardless of whether the technology were used, or even regardless of whether a given hospital owned or had access to a scanner (ProPAC, 1986).

To prevent the potential lag time between cost increase and DRG recalibration, another option would be to adjust immediately the weights of all DRGs that would include cases having undergone MRI. The new weights would be a function of the average additional cost per discharge and the percentage of all cases in each DRG in which MRI was used.

The problem with this alternative, however, is that the patient population to which MRI applies is diverse and difficult to define; MRI scans are done on patients with many different eventual diagnoses, and thus whose cases fall into many different DRGs. It is also possible that MRI might increase costs for some DRGs while lowering costs for others. For these reasons, data on large samples of patients in all relevant DRGs would have to be gathered. Such data are not currently available for MRI patients (ProPAC, 1986).

After dismissing out-of-hand the suggestion that MRI costs be reimbursed on a ''reasonable cost'' basis, thus failing to provide the basic PPS incentive for cost-effective care, ProPAC officials decided upon a final alternative: an additional payment, or add-on, for each MRI scan performed for a Medicare beneficiary. Payments would be directed specifically to those cases in which a scan was performed. Since hospitals with MRI scanners would thus receive higher payments than hospitals without them, adoption and diffusion of this technology would be encouraged; it would become more accessible to Medicare beneficiaries. The lag period associated with recalibration would not be a problem under this alternative; the case-specific nature of this payment would alleviate the problem of higher DRG weights resulting in higher payments when no MRI scan occurred.

The add-on would be calculated according to the average cost of a scan performed at an efficiently run facility. This value was estimated at $335. Because MRI substitutes for a number of other hospital resources, a value of 30% substitution for operating costs and no substitution for capital costs was used to derive an add-on of $124 for institutions with their own scanners and $282 for those that purchase scanners from other providers. Part of the reason for this payment discrepancy is that institutions that own their own scanners qualify for additional reimbursement for capital-related costs under Medicare payment policy (ProPAC, 1986).

The danger in this option is that overpayment may occur as a result of the proposed add-on combining with an increase in DRG weights due to recalibration. It was thus decided that adjustments in DRG weights for MRI would be made for fiscal year 1989, two years after the add-on went into effect. The add-on would be recalculated in fiscal year 1988 and 1989 to adjust for any change in average costs during that time.

The case of magnetic resonance imaging further illustrates the difficulty in fitting new technology into existing categories. A technology such as MRI, capable of diagnosing conditions falling into many different DRGs, does not lend itself easily to federal attempts to categorize neatly disease and its treatment. A similar problem arose with the third new technology we will review here, cochlear implants.

Cochlear Implants

The cochlear implant is a prosthetic device that can assist patients with certain serious forms of hearing impairment. It enhances the ability to detect sounds and speech, improves voice modulation, and increases a hearing-impaired patient's ability to read lips (ProPAC, 1987). The initial FDA approval of cochlear implants involved a single-channel device in 1984. In 1985, an improved multichannel device was introduced and came under consideration for premarketing approval.

Cochlear implants fit into no specific ICD–9 code. They were eventually assigned to DRG 49 (major head and neck procedures), but this decision has been challenged by ProPAC as inappropriate (ProPAC, 1987). ProPAC investigators noted that cochlear implants utilize different resources from other procedures in the same DRG. Many of the procedures in DRG 49 (e.g., glossectomy and laryngectomy) necessitate long lengths of stay and are highly labor intensive. Cochlear implants are much less labor intensive and require shorter lengths of stay.

Moreover, introduction of the more expensive multichannel device brought about a situation where the majority of cochlear implant cases would be underpaid under existing DRG weights, while those cases needing the single-channel device would be overpaid. Average total cost of a single-channel device is $8,550; average total cost of a multichannel device is $14,250; average payment under DRG 49 is $10,000 (ProPAC, 1987).

For these reasons ProPAC analysts reviewed three alternatives to the current DRG classification of cochlear implants:

1. continued assignment to DRG 49;
2. creation of a new DRG for both single- and multichannel devices; or
3. creation of two new DRGs, one for single-channel and one for multichannel devices. (ProPAC, 1987)

ProPAC has recommended that both single- and multichannel implant devices be reassigned to a single new device specific DRG. Although this would most likely result in overpayment for implantation of the single-channel device, it has been noted that 90% of cochlear implants are multichannel: relatively few cochlear implantations would be overpaid under the new classification. In addition, medical indications for each device are clear and well known to physicians; selection of an appropriate cochlear implant would probably not be dictated by financial incentive (ProPAC, 1987).

Because cochlear implants are a new and developing technology, it was recommended that this new DRG be a temporary DRG pending acquisition of sufficient data and experience to understand better the potential of this technology. Consideration for assignment to a permanent DRG would take place within three years of this temporary assignment.

These case studies illustrate some of the complexities and uncertainties involved in fitting new technology into the Prospective Payment System. Arriving at the most equitable and rational alternative, however, does not proceed on a simple case-by-case basis. Federal policy analysts have devised a carefully formulated decision-making process to assist them in cases such as those discussed here. In light of the problems described above, it is informative to gain a more thorough understanding of this process, its strengths, and its limitations.

FITTING A TECHNOLOGY INTO THE PPS SYSTEM: THE FORMAL PROCESS

ProPAC has identified three major questions raised by the problem of adopting new medical and surgical technology under PPS:

1. How might the new hospital and manufacturer incentives under PPS affect the development, adoption, and diffusion of new medical technologies?

2. Are the current PPS mechanisms to create timely and appropriate payments adequate to allow the development, adoption, and diffusion of costly new medical technologies?

3. If current provisions are inadequate, what other mechanisms might be available to encourage the development, adoption, and diffusion of costly new medical technologies? (ProPAC, 1986)

Figure 14.1 illustrates the decision-making process, as developed by ProPAC, involved in the assignment of a new technology to a DRG under PPS. First, agreement must be reached as to whether the new technology is appropriate to an existing DRG category. If so, payment for that category may be adjusted to include use of this new technology. For this to be feasible, the technology must be specific to one DRG or a small group of DRGs. This is not always the case; some technologies are applicable to several DRGs, while others are sufficiently inexpensive that they do not warrant payment adjustment (ProPAC, 1987).

If a technology does not fit into an existing DRG, then a new DRG category may be created for it. Although ProPAC has recommended this for several new technologies such as cochlear implants described above, the only technology-specific DRGs currently in existence apply to heart transplants and multiple major joint procedures of the lower extremity (ProPAC, 1987). HCFA officials, whose responsibility it is to approve recommendations from ProPAC concerning DRG assignments, have expressed concern that the creation of a new DRG category for a particular technology may be the beginning of a return to cost-based reimbursement, and that DRG proliferation will lead to an unwieldy number of DRGs.

To assist in the DRG classification process, ProPAC has developed a set of criteria for assessing whether cases involving a particular technology incur costs significantly different from other cases, and thus whether hospitals offering this technology might be at serious financial risk. If a technology meets enough of the criteria, it might qualify for its own DRG. The criteria are:

1. a significant difference between the dollar amount of cases using the new technology and other cases in the existing DRG;

2. a significant percent dollar difference between cases using the technology and other cases in the DRG;

3. a statistically significant difference between the cost of cases with the technology and the cost of other cases;

4. significant differences in charges between hospitals that adopt the technology and those that do not;

5. significantly greater or less length of stay in cases involving the use of the technology;

6. other major resource use differences (i.e., cost of the technology, use of operating room or ICU);

Figure 14.1
The Decision-Making Process of Classifying and Calculating Payment for New Technologies

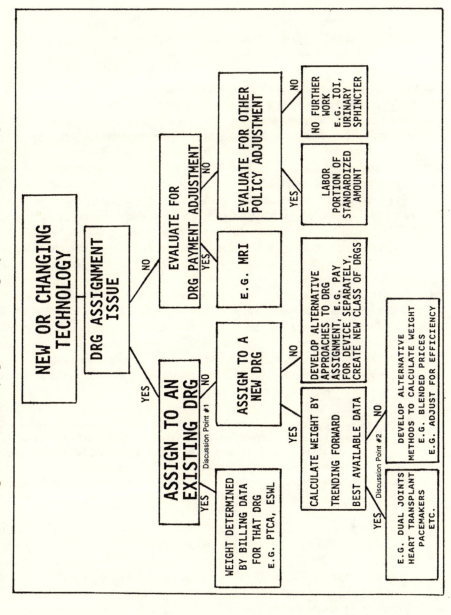

Source: Prospective Payment Assessment Commission, 1987.

7. judgment on the part of ProPAC that cases involving the technology are a distinct subgroup of cases;

8. the new technology being identifiable and discrete;

9. existing evidence that access to the technology will be affected in the absence of payment adjustments; and

10. existing evidence that further development of the technology will be hindered by lack of payment adjustments. (ProPAC, 1987)

Once a technology has been assigned to an existing DRG, it must be decided what data will be used to calculate the payment adjustment needed to include the cost of this new technology. The DRG weight is normally calculated using the best available historical data on costs of the procedure for which the technology is intended.

This method of calculation, however, is not always appropriate. In a case where there is no existing DRG into which a new technology can be fit, historical billing data may be unavailable. Moreover, charges during an early phase of a new technology's implementation may differ substantially from charges later on, due to hospitals becoming more efficient in the technology's use, changes in the way hospitals derive charges and rates, and changes in the manufacturer's price (ProPAC, 1987). The debate on how to classify magnetic resonance imaging illustrates these problems.

When historical data cannot be found or are inappropriate, alternative methods may be used. One such method is price blending. Price blending involves blending an average payment amount with region-specific or hospital type-specific cost data, or with national data from a source other than Medicare's cost data.

Regardless of the method used to calculate DRG weights, the process, as has been seen, can be complex and difficult. ProPAC has developed the following guidelines to assist in these calculations:

The Commission should develop a principle of calculating a weight using the best available data. Criteria should be used to determine when exceptions will be made and when expert judgment will be used to modify the data. Such exceptions should be limited to technologies in early stages of diffusion for which adequate charge or cost data are not available. Where appropriate, experts should be consulted to develop payment amounts that encourage maximum productivity and efficiency. (ProPAC, 1987, 130)

If a new technology cannot be fitted into an existing DRG, there may be alternatives to creating an entire new DRG-specific category for it. In the case of a particularly expensive medical technology devised for use in an already existing procedure, it may be decided that the device should be paid for directly and the rest of the medical procedure should be paid for under an existing DRG. In other cases a new technology may be assigned to a temporary DRG until sufficient cost data are available to make a final decision.

Whichever of these methods is used, it is clear that unforeseen problems can arise to complicate the decision-making process. The fitting of a technology into a DRG for inclusion in PPS, as has been seen, has proved to be more difficult than the architects of PPS had anticipated. As technological innovation continues to blur distinctions such as diagnostic, therapeutic, invasive, and noninvasive, and as new technologies arise that are applicable to a wide variety of cases, problems such as those outlined here can be expected to continue.

SUMMARY AND CONCLUSIONS

PPS was implemented to encourage efficient use of medical procedures and technologies. Under this system, expensive technologies that require long lengths of stay and the extensive use of ancillary services are discouraged. The adoption of ICD–9 codes and the implementation of the DRG classification system, it was hoped, would allow for a rational, easily understood classification scheme to facilitate a distribution of resources that is both equitable and cost efficient.

Nonetheless, as technological research and development continue, policy-makers must grapple with multiple and complex issues as they attempt to fit new forms of medical technology into already established categories. This decision-making process will most likely become even more complex as new technologies are developed. The impact of PPS on the adoption of medical technology is an area requiring intensive research and study. This issue will play an important role in defining the nature of health care in the future.

APPENDIX

Recalibration and updating are the two mechanisms through which technological change can be taken into consideration when changing DRG prices. Updating involves an annual increase or decrease in all prices through utilization of an *update factor*. There are two components to this update factor. The first reflects the level of inflation in the hospital sector (the "hospital market basket"). The second, the discretionary adjustment factor (DAF), accounts for cost changes that may not be captured by measures of inflation, such as those due to changes in quality of care. The DAF reflects ProPAC's judgment concerning the rate at which Medicare standardized amounts should increase or decrease beyond the amount reflected in changes in the hospital market basket. More specifically, the following elements are considered in updating:

1. Changes in composition and prices of goods and services purchased by the hospital (the "hospital market basket");

2. Hospital productivity;

3. Technological and scientific advances;

4. Quality of care provided; and

5. Long-term cost effectiveness in the provision of hospital services.

The update factor can be expressed by the equation:

$$\text{Update} = \text{Market Basket} + \text{DAF}$$

(ProPAC, 1986)

Recalibration of DRG weights, the other available mechanism to take technological change into account, is required by law at least once every four years; ProPAC recommends an annual recalibration because of the rapid change in practice patterns in current volatile, high-technology medical care. Recalibration is the process of adjusting the prices of DRGs relative to each other through changes in DRG weights. A weight is assigned to a DRG according to its assumed resource use in comparison with other DRGs.

The adjustment under recalibration allows a hospital's payment for a patient in a given DRG to stay approximately equal to the cost of treating that patient. Introduction of a new technology can change the cost of treating patients within a given DRG, so this adjustment helps ensure that these new costs will lead to a new price. The manner in which recalibration takes place can thus strongly affect the incentives to adopt new technologies.

There are a number of forms this adjustment can take. "Recalibration," according to ProPAC's definition, includes only the simultaneous adjustment of all DRG weights. If only certain DRG weights are adjusted, the term used is *reweighting*. When all 467 DRGs are recalibrated simultaneously, this is done through empirical reestimation of relative DRG costs. Recalibration may include the creation of new DRGs as a payment mechanism for a particular technology; it may include raising or lowering some DRG weights relative to others to encourage or discourage use of particular technologies within those DRGs.

Also to be noted here are issues concerning the coding of specific cases. As seen in the case of ESWL, the code assigned to a new procedure can determine in which DRG a patient is placed when that procedure is used and can affect the payment a hospital receives for treating that patient.

Until recently, no established mechanism for creating new codes existed, except during the periodic updating of the entire coding system which takes place once every 10 years. Assignment of codes under ICD–9 necessitates consideration of two factors: which code describes the procedure most accurately, and which code will result in an appropriate payment level. ESWL is an example of the type of case in which these two criteria may be conflicting or difficult to define.

There are several problems inherent in the use of ICD–9 as a coding system. Some hospital cases may have been inaccurately classified within DRGs when they were designed, due to inaccurate coding; as a result, some DRG weights may be inaccurate. Moreover, some medical conditions may be described by more than one diagnostic code; this leads to different DRGs with different weights, applicable to the same condition.

There is also a major problem with procedure codes. Current codes may not accurately describe procedures involving new technologies; this confusion can lead to wide variations in DRG assignments. A task force, chaired jointly by the National Center for Health Statistics (NCHS) and the Health Care Financing Administration (HCFA), is currently being established to make coding recommendations and to deal with these discrepancies.

15

Trends in Hospital Capital and the Prospective Payment System: Issues and Implications

Ross M. Mullner

Meeting capital needs is one of the most important issues facing hospitals. Hospitals require adequate infusion of capital to renovate and modernize aging and outdated facilities, respond to changing needs of the communities they serve, provide new services, and purchase new lifesaving and sustaining medical technology.

It has been estimated that during the 1980s, hospitals will need between $100–200 billion in capital to renovate and modernize their facilities (Glenn, 1984, 1). At the same time, however, new economic and political pressures are making it increasingly difficult for hospitals to obtain needed capital.

A multitude of factors make it difficult for hospitals to attract and obtain capital. These include declining admission rates and lengths of stay; growing competition from other hospitals as well as alternative delivery systems (i.e., HMOs, freestanding ambulatory care centers, one-day surgery centers, and home health care organizations); greater numbers of discounted payers; increasing pressure from business, state governments, and the federal government to contain hospital costs; the Gramm-Rudman deficit reduction act; and decreasing Medicare payments for both capital costs and inpatient services.

Another important factor that will have a major impact upon hospitals' ability to access capital as well as their future financing activities is the reform and incorporation of capital costs into Medicare's Prospective Payment System (PPS). At present, Medicare still pays for capital costs on a retrospective cost-based "pass-through" or nonrestrictive basis: interest and depreciation, for example, are subject to virtually no limits and are paid as they are incurred. This payment method, many argue, leads to overinvestment, excess capacity, and higher hospital costs. In 1984, Medicare capital payments totaled $2.9 billion (American Hospital Association, 1986, 2). Congress and the Reagan administration, however, have attempted over the last five years to develop a method to reform capital cost payments and fold them into the Prospective Payment System.

The Reagan administration, Congress, and many health care organizations have developed policy statements and proposals for the reform and incorporation of capital payments. They have tried to address the critical issue of establishing appropriate rates for capital payments with the realization that if rates are set too low, the capital structure, quality, and technology of the hospital industry will deteriorate; conversely, if the rates are set too high, nonprice competition will promote the continued maintenance of excess capital stock and increased costs (Arnould, 1987, 10). Because of the complexity, importance, and possible consequences of reform, no proposal has gained a policy consensus.

It is clear that whatever capital reform policy is enacted will have important long-term implications for hospitals and will influence the quality, cost, and equity of the nation's future health delivery system. As Brown and Saltman (1985, 122) indicate, "Health capital policy is strategically important not only because of the long-term nature of capital commitments but also because capital requirements often drive institutional behavior far out of proportion to dollars expended."

The objective of this chapter is threefold. First, it will review the major trends in sources of hospital capital from the 1920s to the present. Second, it will present an overview of the recent public policy debate of reforming capital payments by folding them into Medicare's Prospective Payment System. Last, it will outline some of the major issues and implications of incorporating hospital capital into the Prospective Payment System.

TRENDS IN SOURCES OF HOSPITAL CAPITAL

Capital financing in the hospital industry has evolved through several major phases over the past decades. There has been a shift away from philanthropy and direct government subsidies toward debt financing and government payments for capital. In the era before the Great Depression, philanthropy was of vital importance. In the era following World War II and preceding Medicare, philanthropic sources were supplemented by direct grants from the federal government. Since Medicare, direct subsidies have diminished and have been replaced by government payments for capital (Cohodes & Kinkead, 1984). However, as the need for capital grew and government assistance did not keep pace, hospitals have increasingly relied on debt financing (American Hospital Association, 1974, 3).

Prior to the Great Depression, a hospital's capital needs were primarily supported through philanthropy from individuals, religious groups, and local government (Bradford, Caldwell & Goldsmith, 1982, 1). In the 1920s, for example, philanthropy provided approximately two-thirds of all capital funds needed by hospitals (Laffey & Lappen, 1976). With the Great Depression and until the end of World War II, however, capital investment in the hospital industry was at a virtual standstill.

Although philanthropy as a funding source continued to increase in absolute dollars throughout the post–World War II period, as a percentage of total hospital capital it has declined dramatically. In 1973, for example, philanthropy accounted for 10% of funding sources for hospital construction; in 1981 it had declined to 4% (Elrod & Wilkinson, 1985, 4). The reasons for this decline are not clear, but they seem to include inflation (Elrod & Wilkinson, 1985, 4); the increase in the sheer size and rapidity of growth in hospital capital spending; the incorporation of local businesses into larger national and international conglomerates that may have led to decreased concern with local communities; the increasing weariness of some contributors to invest further in communities; and the greater involvement of the federal government in paying for health facilities and services (Kinkead, 1984, 57).

A second major phase of capital financing began with the enactment of the federal Hospital Survey and Construction Act of 1946, better known as the Hill-Burton program. This program, which provided grants to states to develop state-wide plans for the construction of hospital facilities and to assist in the construction of such facilities, was established in response to the rapid technological advances in medicine as well as to the heightened postwar awareness concerning access to health care. Also, because of the lack of investment in hospital facilities during the depression and the years of World War II, it was generally held that a shortage of community hospital beds existed, particularly in rural areas.

In 1970, the Hill-Burton program was converted from a grant to a loan and loan guarantee program. Fiscal pressures on both federal and state governments to balance their budgets and reduce health care expenditures contributed to the curtailment of capital grant programs in the early 1970s. In 1973, Hill-Burton loans were reduced to one-third of the previous year's volume, forcing hospitals to increase their reliance on debt markets for financing capital projects. The Hill-Burton program finally ended in the late 1970s.

During the life of the program, Hill-Burton provided approximately $4 billion in grants to nearly 4,000 hospitals and $1.9 billion in loan and loan guarantees to almost 300 hospitals (U.S. General Accounting Office, 1982). As one author (Shaw, 1985, 17) summarized the results of the program: "The Hill-Burton Act of 1946 disbursed few strings attached monies from the federal government to build or reconstruct hospitals. As a result, unparalleled bed growth occurred between 1950 and 1970. Approximately 350,000 hospital beds were constructed. That is about one-third of today's total community hospital bed population."

The next major phase of capital financing began with the growth of private health insurance and the implementation of the Medicare and Medicaid programs. The growth of Blue Cross plans and other private health insurance, due in part to the rapid growth of employee fringe-benefit packages, greatly expanded the role of third-party payers as a source of hospital revenue.

In particular, Blue Cross greatly expanded during the post–World War II period. For example, in 1937 there were 37 Blue Cross plans with 1 million members. In 1947, the total membership had grown to 27 million, or 19% of the U.S. population. By 1958, there were 79 plans with 52 million members, equivalent to 30% of the U.S. population (Berman, Weeks & Kukla, 1986, 142).

In the mid–1960s, the federal government established the Medicare and Medicaid programs. These programs shifted the role of the federal government from financing buildings and equipment to purchasing hospital services for the elderly and the poor.

It is interesting to note that much of the negotiations in 1965 and 1966 between the federal government and the hospital industry centered on capital reimbursement. Most of the hospital industry's demands were met. This was partly because the industry was successful in making government policymakers believe there was a capital shortage and partly because policymakers wanted to imbue hospitals with enthusiasm for the program (Kinkead, 1984, 50).

The growth of private health insurance and the establishment of Medicare and Medicaid were significant for several reasons. They increased the number of patients treated at hospitals, increasing hospital revenues and adding financial stability to hospitals' cash flow. They established cost-reimbursement methods that recognized depreciation and interest as reimbursable expenses. They were generous in providing reimbursement for new services, which meant hospitals could purchase new medical equipment and technology and be virtually assured of their costs in doing so. And they laid the financial foundation for hospitals to borrow funds from capital markets for financing capital projects based on anticipated future revenues.

The fourth major phase of capital financing started in the late 1960s and early to mid–1970s with the enactment of legislation by many states allowing hospitals to issue tax-exempt revenue bonds through state and/or local bodies. Although not much has been written on their legislative origins, it appears that the Connecticut Health and Educational Facility Authority was the first to implement such financing in 1966. This was followed by New York (1970), New Jersey (1973), and Illinois (1974) and many other states (Metz, 1983, 4).

This major phase of capital financing had little public debate and little concern with how it would impact upon other state and federal policies. According to Kinkead (1984, 61):

It is one of the ironies of modern health financing policy that perhaps the most important reform affecting hospital capital formation sprang not from the federal government or Congress, but from state legislatures. It is also ironic that the reform appears to have occurred with little public debate or with little concern for how tax-exempt financing might affect the other policy objectives of state governments (such as certificate-of-need regulation) or the policy objectives of the federal government (for example, cost containment in the federal insurance program).

Tax-exempt financing has several major advantages to hospitals. First, tax-exempt bonds open a vast new pool of capital to hospitals: the public money markets and tax-exempt bond buyers. Second, tax-exempt financing makes it easier for hospitals to provide security for loans. Debt can be secured with the pledge of future revenue and the guarantee of federal mortgage insurance. Third, the bond market offers hospitals flexibility in terms of debt payment schedules. Fourth, the lower but tax-exempt interest rates make the debt coverage requirement of lenders easier to meet. Fifth, interest expense is a fully reimbursable cost under Medicare, Medicaid, and cost-based Blue Cross plans (Kinkead, 1984, 62–63).

Several federal laws were enacted in the 1960s and 1970s that in turn helped states establish debt financing mechanisms for hospitals. In 1963, IRS Revenue Ruling 63–20 permitted not-for-profit hospitals to issue tax-exempt bonds through a municipality under the condition that ownership of the facility be turned over to the city or county when the bonds were retired. In 1968, Section 242 was added to the National Housing Act. Section 242 authorized the Federal Housing Administration to provide mortgage insurance for loans to private, not-for-profit hospitals, and later to for-profit hospitals. This insurance covered construction loans as well as loans to purchase major movable equipment for hospitals. In 1974, the federal government enacted P. L. 92–419 which provided rural health facilities with loans through the Farmer's Home Administration (National Health Lawyer's Association, 1982).

The increase in hospital debt financing was further influenced by high rates of inflation in the 1970s. Long-term interest rates were consistently less than inflation rates, resulting in borrowers paying back loans with dollars worth less than those originally borrowed. Inflation may also have served to reduce the number of philanthropic dollars as a percentage of total funding sources. In 1973, debt financing accounted for 64% of funding sources for hospital construction; in 1981 it increased to 69% (Elrod & Wilkinson, 1985, 4).

In the 1980s, debt financing has continued to be the most important source of capital for hospitals. State and local mechanisms have become the predominant means to issue hospital tax-exempt bonds. At present, 27 states have state authorities and 34 states have legislation enabling other governmental units to issue hospital tax-exempt bonds (Moss, 1988). In 10 states, hospitals can elect to sell tax-exempt bonds through either a state or local authority (Metz, 1983, 4).

However, it appears that many hospitals are finding capital more difficult to obtain. Because of recent declines in admission rates and lengths of stay, increasing competition, greater numbers of discounted payers, decreasing Medicare payments for both capital costs and for inpatient services, and the uncertainty of how capital costs will be reformed and folded into the Prospective Payment System, hospital credit ratings have declined, and interest rates for long-term debt have increased (Bruton & Waterman, 1985, 38).

THE DEBATE OVER CAPITAL REFORM AND THE
PROSPECTIVE PAYMENT SYSTEM

Researchers and public-policy analysts have increasingly recognized the problematic effects of cost-based reimbursement for capital and hospital operating costs. Brown and Saltman (1985, 126), for example, write:

Because capital purchases become essentially cost free to investing institutions in good financial health, cost-based reimbursement encourages overinvestment in equipment and capacity and excessive reliance on debt financing. Moreover, because reimbursement for depreciation exceeds loan principle payments in the early years of a loan, capital investment under retrospective reimbursement principles generates cash flow windfalls for hospitals and encourages periodic refinancing rather than retirement of debt. Standard reimbursement rules also foster hospital acquisition because acquisition-related costs are fully reimbursable.

Capital use also is stimulated by cost-based mechanisms for reimbursement of hospital operating expenses. By guaranteeing payment for most operating costs associated with capital investment, cost-based reimbursement systems encourage overexpansion of facilities and services. Overexpansion, in turn, increases overall system operating costs because utilization tends to rise to fill existing capacity. A costly spiral of investment and utilization results.

In 1983, Congress attempted to address some of the problems of retrospective cost-based reimbursement. It enacted legislation to change Medicare's reimbursement methods. Specifically, Congress, using diagnosis-related groups (DRGs), enacted the Medicare Prospective Payment System for hospital operating costs.

Congress, however, delayed any action on the prospective payment of capital costs. It kept in place Medicare's method of reimbursing hospitals for capital costs on a retrospective cost-based basis. At the same time, Congress directed the secretary of the Department of Health and Human Services (HHS) to develop a proposal in one year (October 1, 1984) to reform and fold capital costs into the Prospective Payment System. Because of a mix of political, technical, and circumstantial events, HHS took three years to develop the proposal, which it submitted to Congress in 1986 (American Hospital Association, 1986).

From 1983 to 1986, many different groups, including the hospital industry, investment bankers, equipment manufacturers, hospital financial managers, and health planners developed positions and policies regarding the reform and incorporation of capital costs into PPS under Medicare. In addition, proposals were developed by Congress (e.g., Sen. Durenberger and Sen. Quayle, Bill S. 1559, [1985]) and the administration as to how these payments should be made. The differences among these proposals primarily centered on such items as capping the capital payment add-on to each DRG, separating the treatment of moveable equipment from that for fixed assets, and the length and the timing of the prospective payment phase-in or transition period.

The debate in Congress in 1986 failed to yield a resolution as to the best approach for incorporating capital. At that point, Congress decided to continue the cost pass-through method of payment for capital for at least one more year but at reduced payment levels. This was passed as part of the Omnibus Budget Reconciliation Act of 1986 (OBRA–1986). According to this act, allowable Medicare hospital inpatient capital-related payments were to be reduced by 3.5% in FY 1987, by 7% in FY 1988, and by 10% in FY 1989.

In passing OBRA–1986, Congress indicated its intent to pass legislation incorporating capital into PPS prices by FY 1988. However, in the event that Congress did not exercise its prerogative to legislate on this matter, it recognized the secretary's authority, beginning in FY 1988, to incorporate capital into PPS prices through regulation. Congress, however, prohibited the secretary from issuing final regulations until September 1, 1987, giving Congress the time and opportunity to act first. Congress also stipulated in the act that the secretary's capital incorporation approach must be consistent with the budget goals specified in OBRA–1986.

In 1987, no formal legislative proposals to incorporate capital into PPS prices were introduced into Congress. The administration, however, published in the Federal Register proposed regulations for capital incorporation on May 19, 1987, and final regulations on September 1, 1987.

The regulations were to be effective for hospital cost reporting periods beginning on or after October 1, 1987. They split capital costs into two components: plant and fixed equipment and moveable equipment.

Plant and fixed equipment were to be incorporated into PPS over a 10-year transition period. In the first year of the transition, 95% of a hospital's actual plant/fixed costs would be paid retrospectively, as under the old system, with the remaining 5% reimbursed according to a fixed federal amount. The second-year blend would be 90% hospital-specific and 10% federal, with the following years having percent blends of 85/15, 80/20, 75/25, 70/30, 60/40, 50/50, 35/65, and 20/80. A 100% federal rate was to be achieved by October 1, 1997. The rate would differ between urban and rural hospitals, with urban institutions paid at a higher rate due to higher construction costs.

For moveable equipment, capital costs were to be incorporated over a seven-year transition period. The transition follows the schedule for plant/fixed equipment for the first four years at 95/5, 90/10, 85/15, and 80/20. In the fifth year, the proportions were to become 70/30; in the sixth, 50/50; and in the seventh, 25/75. A 100% federal rate was to be achieved by October 1, 1994.

Congress, however, overrode the regulations by enacting budget bill P. L. 100–203. Under this law, Medicare capital payments were cut 12% as of January 1, 1988, and 15% in FY 1989. Also, it restricted HHS from folding hospital capital costs into PPS until FY 1992 (Sorian, 1987, 1).

At present, it does not seem likely that the administration or Congress will attempt to address capital reform in the near future. It seems very likely, however, that they will continue to derive policy through decremental budgeting and across-the-board funding cuts. This approach will likely lower hospitals' ability to attract capital, reduce expenditures for plant and equipment, and continue the uncertainty of starting new hospital construction and renovation projects and purchasing new medical equipment and technology.

ISSUES AND IMPLICATIONS OF CAPITAL REFORM

Although it is clear that capital reform and its incorporation into the Medicare PPS will have important effects upon hospitals, it is not obvious or easy to determine what these effects will be. Much will depend upon the rate of capital cost payments; the age of the facility, its equipment, and technology; the type of patients and services provided by the institution; and the type of hospital (i.e., voluntary, for-profit, or state or local government owned; member of a multihospital system or a stand-alone facility; a major research, teaching, or non-teaching hospital) and its capital needs.

In terms of rate of payment and the age of the facility, Arnould & DeBrock (1986, 276–77) point out:

If the capital cost payment to hospitals is set too low, it penalizes hospitals with high capital costs, possibly to the extent of exclusion from the market. Unfortunately, these high costs may have resulted from recent renovation projects designed to increase efficiency and reduce costs, such as expanded outpatient surgery facilities. At the same time, low allowances for capital costs may protect hospitals with older and possibly less efficient physical plants. Similarly, unreasonably low payments could discourage other hospitals with older plants and concomitant low capital costs from undertaking capital improvement projects which would increase efficiency, even if these hospitals have high occupancy levels.

If the payments for capital costs are set too high, two effects could occur. First, they might not provide any incentive to reduce the excess capacity which clearly exists in the industry. Second, an Averch-Johnson effect might result [Averch & Johnson, 1962]. The Averch-Johnson model, developed to analyze the nature of capital formation in regulated public utilities, predicts that, where the allowed rate of return on capital is greater than the cost of capital, firms have an incentive to overcapitalize. Thus, excessive reimbursements for capital could lead to inefficient expansion of capacity (in the case of hospitals, a lack of contraction) in an industry already plagued by excess capacity.

In terms of types of hospitals and the patients they serve, Brown and Saltman state (1985, 128) that the repeal of Medicare retrospective cost-based reimbursement of capital "may exclude most voluntary hospitals from access to private capital for major replacement and renovation," and that it will accelerate "the competitive advantages enjoyed by corporate delivery systems and exacerbate existing differentials in racial and class access to adequate care and facilities."

One can conjecture that voluntary hospitals, freestanding hospitals (not members of multihospital systems), large urban teaching hospitals, and small rural hospitals seem likely to feel the adverse impact of capital reform.

Because voluntary hospitals rely extensively upon tax-exempt bond financing, they seem likely to have greater difficulty in attracting new financing with major changes in capital payments. With major changes, their bonds may not be attractive to buyers.

Freestanding hospitals may have a more difficult time attracting capital. It has been argued that hospitals in multihospital systems with their greater assets have higher bond ratings (Hernandez & Howie, 1979) and attract capital at lower rates (Ermann & Gabel, 1984). With capital reform, hospitals not in a multihospital system may experience more problems in attracting capital.

Large teaching hospitals that have a major commitment to medical education and research will also likely have a more difficult time attracting capital. These hospitals may find it increasingly difficult to purchase new, expensive medical technology.

Last, small rural hospitals with their large proportion of Medicare patients would also seem likely to be adversely affected by capital reform. Many of these facilities, which are old and in need of renovation and replacement, may find it difficult to attract capital.

SUMMARY AND CONCLUSION

This chapter has attempted to present the major trends in the sources of hospital capital from the 1920s to the present—identifying how they have changed and the underlying sources of those changes. It has shown there has been a marked shift away from philanthropy and direct government subsidies toward government payments for capital and a tremendous growth of debt financing.

The problematic effects of Medicare's retrospective cost-based method of reimbursement—overinvestment in equipment and capacity and excessive reliance on debt financing and the overexpansion of facilities and services—were discussed. An overview of the recent five-year public policy debate by the Reagan administration, Congress, and various health care groups over the reform of capital payments and its incorporation into the Medicare Prospective Payment System was provided. Because of the complexity of the issues and the inability to obtain a consensus, Congress is postponing capital reform for hospitals for several years.

Finally, this chapter has tried to present the important issues and implications of reforming hospital capital costs. It is clear that whatever capital reform policy is enacted in the future, it will have a major impact upon hospitals. A number of key questions will need to be addressed: Will the reform and new rates of capital cost payments lead to increases in hospital closure? Will it mean the end of health planning and certificate-of-need programs? What will be the impact on hospitals with a large number of Medicaid patients? Will inner-city hospitals, rural hospitals, and hospitals with teaching and research programs be differentially affected? What will be the impact on for-profit and voluntary hospitals, on hospitals in multihospital systems and hospitals that are freestanding? What will happen to the rate of technological diffusion, and therefore accessibility to new technology? Will hospitals lack the funds to purchase new and needed technology?

Clearly, the problems and changes that will occur with hospital capital reform will provide many managerial, public policy, and health services research questions for the future.

ACKNOWLEDGMENTS

The author is grateful to Donna J. Melkonian, American Hospital Association, Barry S. Maram, Illinois Health Facilities Authority, and Dr. Richard J. Arnould, University of Illinois, for their substantial input and assistance in the preparation of this chapter.

16

The Effects of a Competitive Health Care Environment on the Adoption of Medical Technology

Mary P. Taggart and David T. Griffin

The health care industry has changed greatly during the last 10 years. A decade ago the key issues for the industry centered mainly upon regulation and control. In 1974, certificate-of-need (CON) legislation gave state-designated agencies the power to reject hospital decisions to build, expand, or modernize their physical plants or expend more than some designated amount on new equipment. By 1976 there were CON laws in 24 states and similar legislation in 7 others. Furthermore, the National Health Planning and Resources Development Act (1974) extended the authorization of CON programs to all states.

Ten years later, the concern shifted to economic incentives and payment restrictions to control the amounts paid for health care by Medicare and other intermediaries. As a result of Medicare's new Prospective Payment System (PPS), hospitals and other health care providers currently compete for limited resources. What has actually developed post-PPS is a competitive environment in which all parties involved have strong economic incentives to maximize profits. Hospitals and physicians now have greater incentives to encourage quicker adoption of expensive yet profitable technologies in their institutions and are increasingly finding that technology can create new competitive opportunities.

The objective of this chapter is to discuss the interaction between technology and competition. Specifically, the first section will discuss the process of technology adoption and diffusion. The next section will discuss the changing competitive health care environment brought about by the shift to cost containment and PPS. The last section will tie these two areas together and discuss the implications for new medical technology.

TECHNOLOGY ADOPTION AND DIFFUSION

When we think of medical technology we often think of major, costly, sophisticated medical equipment. We think of such recent technologies as computed tomography (CT) scanning and magnetic resonance imaging (MRI). Although many new medical technologies are not as well known nor as costly as these two, all medical technologies have underlying them a medical procedure. A procedure ordered by a physician may be either diagnostic or therapeutic. A major capital investment may be required in order to deliver the procedure; in some cases, conversely, only consumable costs may be associated with it.

In understanding how medical technology is adopted and diffused, it is necessary to understand the medical procedure behind it. In general, we believe that the constructs of adoption theory as put forth by Rogers (1983) are applicable to medical markets and technology. If one studies the roles of various procedures and how they will be used in different circumstances, one will find a fairly predictable pattern in the diffusion of medical technology. The key to understanding the process is to understand the relative utility of various procedures and how relative utility changes over time.

Figure 16.1 shows the relationship between the cumulative adoption curve and various stages in the development of medical technology. The figure shows that long before any new procedure is performed or any new equipment is purchased, there is basic research. This research is conducted without a specific hypothesis to test. This stage is followed by more detailed applied research where there is generally a hypothesis to test. Further, the hypothesis may suggest the potential value it is going to have. Next, the investigator may conduct clinical investigations to prove the safety and efficacy of the procedure or technology. This clinically applied research is often part of the Food and Drug Administration approval process. At this point there has been some limited use on an actual patient population. Once this stage has passed, others in the medical community will attempt to replicate the results of the clinical investigations and begin a debate about the relative utility of the new technology or procedure. During the next stage of adoption, the early adopters begin to evaluate the technology and, assuming it has positive utility, the market begins to develop.

Figure 16.2 shows the normal adoption pattern of an innovation as derived from adoption theory. For the first use of a new procedure or the first purchase of a new piece of technology you tend to see a bell-shaped frequency curve of adopters over time. First, a small group of individuals or institutions known as the innovators will put the new technology to test. This group will be among the first to experiment with the new technology specifically for clinical application on a patient population base. Teaching hospitals are usually the innovators in attempts to gain prestige or to attract leading researchers to their institutions.

Figure 16.1
Cumulative Adoption: The *S* Curve

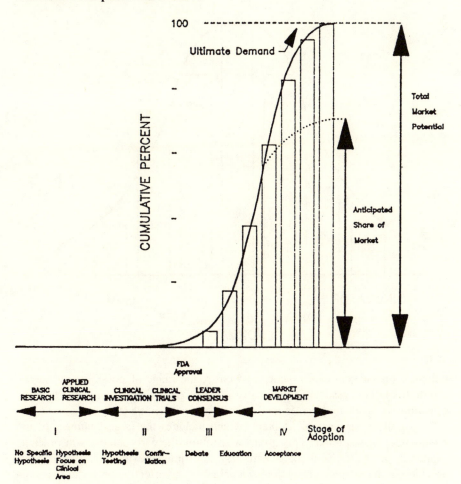

This was typical for technologies such as cardiac nuclear imaging where the utility of the procedure for the patient was not clear. These teaching institutions provide valuable data on this procedure and the related equipment; however, the application of the information is rather limited for further development in non-teaching hospitals (Pozen et al., 1984).

As time continues, the next group to adopt the new technology is the early adopters. This group will take the new technology along with the innovators' experience and implement it for the initial purpose of attracting patients. If this group is successful in doing so, it will have a greater chance of dominating the market. However, "in the wake of rapid technical evolution and its considerable

Figure 16.2
Normal Adoption Pattern

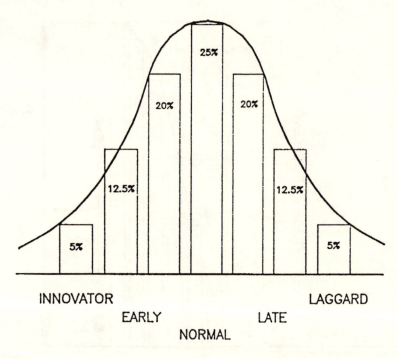

INNOVATOR   LAGGARD
                    EARLY   LATE
                              NORMAL

influence on medical care practice and costs, the range of possible advantages and disadvantages associated with early adoption of any technology, particularly of cardiac nuclear imaging, is unclear'' (Pozen et al., 1984).

Next will be the normal adopters (which includes the largest number of individuals or institutions). This group will follow the early adopters in order to capture a piece of the market share. By this time, the technology has been accepted in the medical profession as a valuable and effective procedure. Therefore, by concentrating on strong marketing efforts, this group should be able to create demand for the technology in a profitable manner.

The late adopters and laggards are those groups that remained pessimistic of the profitable value during the technology's development. As a result, they wait until most of the competition has accepted the new technology before investing their resources. The risk of investment at this time is much lower; however, this group will have less of a market potential than the earlier adopters.

Figure 16.3 shows the competitive strategies of early and late developers of a medical technology. Those companies that elect to enter into the early development stage of a new technology follow a very high-risk–high-return strategy. They may, in effect, define a new market. If they are successful they will be the early leaders and will have the greatest chance of dominating the market. In

Figure 16.3
Marketplace Entry Strategies

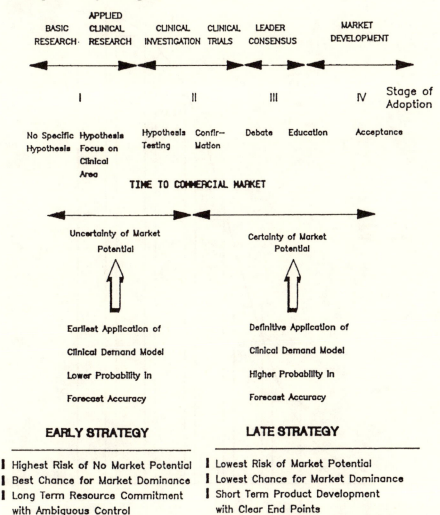

contrast, those companies that elect to enter into the late-development stage of a new technology follow a lower-risk–lower-return strategy. They must concentrate on product enhancement and marketing in order to take shares from the leader.

Figure 16.4 shows the *s*-shaped cumulative adoption curve of an innovation

Figure 16.4
Cumulative Adoption Curve

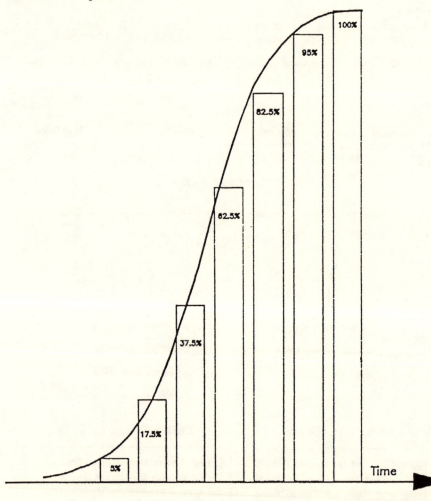

over time. This curve rises slowly as the innovators and a small portion of the early adopters begin the process of diffusion. Then the curve rises sharply as the early and normal adopters begin anxiously to acquire the innovation. It then increases at a gradually slower rate as the few remaining laggards finally adopt. This type of curve may be used to describe the cumulative adoption of a new medical technology.

When an innovative procedure or piece of equipment becomes available, hospitals and other health care providers must decide upon their market strategy. Much like the companies that provide the products, they need to decide whether they want to be innovators or early adopters or wait until a new technology is proven. This is an increasingly important part of a provider's definitive market strategy.

To illustrate, one recent technology that has had a long history of experimental development and change is percutaneous transluminal coronary angioplasty. This procedure originally consisted of inserting a balloon catheter into a coronary artery and inflating it to reduce the amount of obstruction. The first percutaneous transluminal angioplasty was performed in January 1964. However, it was not until May 1977, 13 years later, before the first percutaneous transluminal coronary angioplasty was actually performed on a patient as part of bypass surgery. Six months later, in September 1977, it was first performed in a cardiac catheterization laboratory. The procedure was first performed in the United States in March 1978. After its approval by the Food and Drug Administration it was widely adopted. The next major change in the procedure occurred in 1983 when the first laser angioplasty was performed.

Another example illustrates the diffusion of CT procedures. Figure 16.5 illustrates the annualized volume of CT head procedures in the nation for the period 1972–90, as forecasted in 1977, long before the advent of MRI. Since the procedure was first introduced in 1972, the number of procedures greatly increased as forecasted. Thus, this procedure exhibited the classic characteristics of the s-shaped cumulative adoption curve. It is now being partially displaced by MRI.

Figure 16.6 shows the cumulative penetration of ultrasound by U.S. hospitals in various bed-size groups for the period 1972–81. This figure clearly shows the s-shaped curves for the larger-size hospitals, especially for those in the 300- to 500-bed-size categories. The figure also shows that larger-size hospitals were more likely to adopt ultrasound and that innovative intensity appears to be directly correlated to the bed size of the hospitals. Lastly, the figure shows that after ultrasound was first introduced to hospitals in the early 1970s, by the early 1980s large hospitals had almost fully adopted the technology. In contrast, smaller hospitals were still in the early adoption stage with respect to ultrasound.

At this point we move away from a discussion of examples and into the key forecasting elements that can alter the shape of the cumulative adoption curve discussed previously (Figure 16.7). The history of a technology's research and assessment (point 1) determines when that particular procedure will be first introduced in a health care institution. After being introduced, a number of early innovators will begin to adopt it (point 2). At this time, it is still unclear how far the innovation will diffuse into the medical environment. What will determine the potential impact of the innovation is the level of ultimate demand (point 4 or 4'). This may be either high (point 4') or low (point 4) depending on the clinical role a procedure will fulfill, the size of the relevant patient population, and the cost. In addition, regulation, payment systems, and competition will affect ultimate demand. An example was illustrated by Hillman and Schwartz (1985) in their discussion of the differences between CT scanners and MRI diffusion (Figure 16.8). As shown in the figure, the MRI diffusion lagged behind

Figure 16.5
1979–1990 Head CT Procedures: Forecast vs. Actual

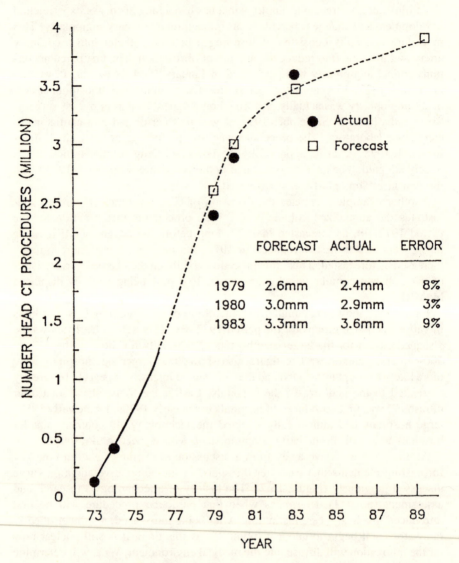

	FORECAST	ACTUAL	ERROR
1979	2.6mm	2.4mm	8%
1980	3.0mm	2.9mm	3%
1983	3.3mm	3.6mm	9%

the pace set by the CT during the first years of clinical availability. For example, over 400 CT units were installed within the first four years of diffusion compared to 151 MRI units. The reasons behind this difference are largely due to cost and relative clinical utility. Other reasons include Medicare's Prospective Payment System, CON regulation, and competitive market forces in existence during the development of MRI.

Figure 16.6
Cumulative Penetration of Any Ultrasound in Hospital Radiology Departments

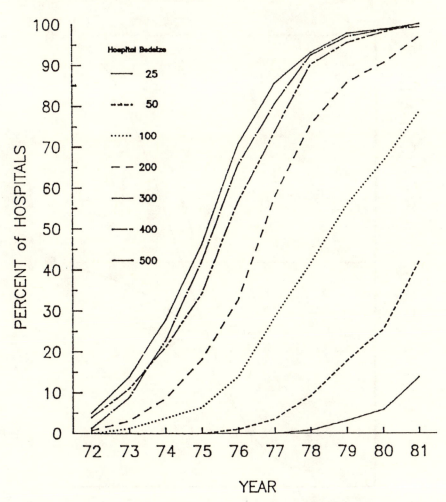

THE COMPETITIVE ENVIRONMENT AND TECHNOLOGY ADOPTION

An analysis of the adoption process requires attention to the role of the current competitive health care environment. This competitive environment is based on three situations: competition among payers, competition among providers, and competition among suppliers of health care technology. Each entity, in its own way, is attempting to maximize its financial position by the function of its market or cost position: they are either controlling their costs or increasing their market share in order to compete profitably with others in the market. What is unique

Figure 16.7
Key Forecasting Elements

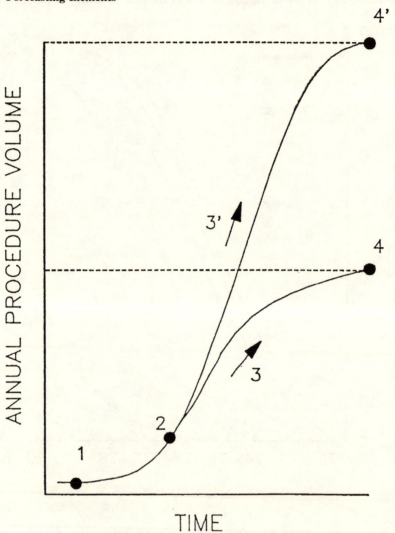

about the health care industry is that each one of these entities is interrelated. They depend on the development of each other in order to survive.

For example, suppliers want hospitals (providers) to adopt their new equipment. At the same time, hospitals want the payers to reimburse them for the procedures performed with the new equipment. However, post-PPS payers only want to reimburse those procedures that are least costly and most efficient. If

Figure 16.8
**The Diffusion of CT and MRI since the Introduction of the First Clinical Human
Imaging Prototype in the United States (CT, June 1973; MRI, December 1980)**

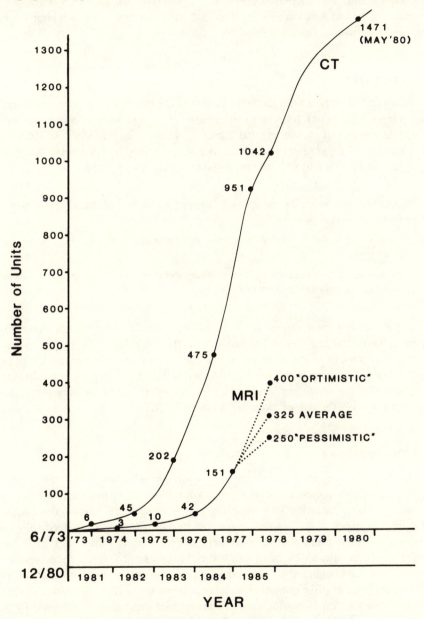

Source: Hillman & Schwartz, 1985. Reprinted with permission.

the equipment does not meet these criteria, the payers will not likely reimburse the provider. Providers not getting paid for the service will not, therefore, demand the equipment. The increased pressures of payers in the post-PPS era and the increasing cost to develop new technologies have resulted in a much higher level of interdependence among these three entities.

The Payers

In order to compete with the other payers in the health care market, each must keep rates low enough to attract subscribers yet high enough to cover expenses; limit the number of encounters that subscribers have with providers; and increase the number of subscribers to each of its particular health care plans. However, in order to do this and still maximize profits, each payer must:

1. Select favorable subscriber groups (i.e., attract patients who are least likely to require expensive medical attention).
2. Use price pressures to control payments per encounter (i.e., use copayments and deductibles).
3. Develop utilization controls to control encounters per subscriber (i.e., use second opinions, use only selected providers).

By increasing their efforts with utilization controls and price pressures, the payers have changed their relationship with the providers. The providers have accepted a variety of these elements, such as fixed payments per service or per patient or prospective-based payment. As a result, these changes have influenced the styles of the providers by forcing them to utilize fewer services per patient and to optimize the use of essential services.

The Providers

In this new competitive environment, each provider has found that it must attract profitable patients, create referral networks, select profitable services to deliver, choose lucrative technologies, and offer services beyond the original facility. In order to do this and maximize profits, the providers need to select favorable patients and provide profitable services. In addition, they must also minimize expenditures by minimizing variable costs per service, reducing overhead, and lengthening the replacement cycles on the technology they adopt. Providers need to offer profitable services in order to survive. A number of these services depend on technological innovations that must also be accepted by the payers in order to be reimbursed. In addition, these providers do not want unreliable equipment or equipment that will become obsolete a short time after being purchased; they want it around long enough to yield a return on investment.

The Suppliers

The suppliers of medical equipment are facing various forces in the competitive environment. The first is price pressure. This stems directly from the providers wanting to keep purchasing costs down, and indirectly from payers wanting less-expensive and less-resource-intensive services from providers. In addition, the payers also encounter price pressures from their competitors which means that each must develop an effective pricing strategy.

Secondly, suppliers face volume pressure. As providers attempt to decrease use of the product, volume goes down for the supplier.

Thirdly, the suppliers encounter high risks. They become less certain of the return on the resources (mainly capital) invested in their innovations; therefore, they are betting mostly on what they believe to be sure winners. This uncertainty will most likely prohibit the development of questionable technologies as well as some that could ultimately prove highly beneficial.

Finally, the suppliers' research and development departments confront pressures to focus on "sure winners" early on in the development of technology. This often leads to joint ventures with scientists and researchers for innovative ideas. By doing this the suppliers hope to end up with less of a financial commitment. Examples of this occurred in the development of cardiac care units (CCUs). Warner-Lambert Pharmaceuticals and Hewlett-Packard participated and supported the research, development, and promotion of CCUs because the technology that would eventually equip these units was manufactured by these corporations (Siegel, 1987).

Implications of the Competitive Health Care Environment for Technology Adoption

The three major entities of the competitive health care environment are seeking a symbiotic relationship in which all three "win." The suppliers want to produce a profitable product or service that is demanded by the providers. The providers want the new technology because it attracts patients or minimizes costs. In addition, the payers will reimburse the providers who purchase this equipment because it limits the encounters with providers or reduces the cost per encounter. When this "win-win-win" situation occurs, the new technology will make an impact in the health care environment.

The pressures applied by payers and providers elicit different strategic responses depending on the type of product and its position on the diffusion curve. In the following, we describe four strategic responses pertinent to today's environment.

PRICE STRATEGIES

For mature products where technological development and improvements have almost ceased, suppliers are left to compete largely on the basis of price. PPS increased price pressure significantly. Suppliers must also concentrate on selling their products in high volume across many product lines. Long-term price discounts and bundling are used to provide savings to the providers who purchase the product and induce them to remain loyal to the supplier. These strategies are developed because the mature products have substitute goods present in the market to compete against. Also, because these are mature products, the supplier often does not have alternative strategies except for divestiture or value adding. This situation is largely a win-win-lose where suppliers lose. Examples include X-ray film, IV solutions, generic drugs, and surgical supplies.

Value-Added Strategy

Rather than compete solely on price, suppliers of mature products in recent years have attempted to add value to the product. This entails making it easier or faster for a customer to obtain or use the product. This usually involves reducing the amount of labor needed to prepare, deliver, or monitor a product. Suppliers can increase revenue by substituting a product for labor and/or reducing labor skills required to use a product. In today's environment, where labor costs are of great concern and where skilled labor shortages are increasingly common, this can be a win-win-win strategy. If the product provides a net positive added value, then the current PPS system favors its adoption. Examples include automatic controllers on IV solutions, bar coding on laboratory instruments, unit dose on pharmacy products, and computerized interpretation of Holter Monitors.

Product Strategies

Following the introduction of new technology and its movement into early adoption, the number of competitors increases rapidly. What follows is a product development race. There are four key dimensions of development—efficacy, cost, risk, and speed/ease of use. While the "ideal" is instantaneous 100% efficacy at no risk or cost to the patient, no product comes near this ideal. Product improvement along each dimension faces the law of diminishing returns: the cost of developing an improvement increases exponentially, and the value of the improvement decreases similarly. The current environment rewards improvement in each dimension independently. However, most product developments entail trade-offs, greater efficacy at higher cost, lower risk at higher cost, and so on.

With numerous suppliers pursuing individual strategies, each of which has a different emphasis among the four dimensions, it is difficult to predict who the winner(s) will be. Most medical technologies have witnessed turbulent changes in market leadership during the period of early to normal adoption. One develops a short-term advantage only to be displaced by another. Examples are numerous, including CT, ultrasound, and chemistry and immunochemistry. Seldom does a single company pace developments over an extended period; Coulter in hematology is a rare example.

The period of product development is exciting to witness, but it has few winners. Providers face a perplexing array of choices and feel more competitive and economic pressures to make the right choice. However, PPS makes it difficult for providers to adopt a new product for which cost is higher even if it performs better. DRGs are not quickly adjusted to incorporate their costs and benefits. Suppliers' fortunes thus rise and fall. At the end of the process, the consumer wins as the technology settles down along its optimal configuration.

"Redefining the Game" Strategy

Earlier in Figure 16.3 we reviewed supplier strategy as it related to technology development. Those who got in early on a technology's development (long before market) bear a high risk with a potential for high return. This has long been the lure of the medical products market. Many new technologies have truly been revolutionary—they redefined the game in terms of how a given clinical situation was diagnosed or treated.

Initially, most breakthroughs added a capability where none existed before. The alternative was that the patient went undiagnosed or untreated. When introduced, these products added to the high cost of medical care and became the scapegoats for health care inflation. Their use was often regulated by CON. Examples include cardiac catheterization/open heart surgery, patient monitoring, artificial joints, transplants, pacemakers, and CT scanners. To the degree that they reduced cost, it was over the long run and to the entire health system. However, these technologies created huge, new markets and many new suppliers. Such new products face a tougher test today. Market development takes longer and is riskier.

In the 1980s, most "redefining the game" opportunities have recognized the need to displace an established, expensive procedure or product. In effect, the breakthroughs can reduce cost, improve performance, reduce risk, and save time. The current environment favors these as the real win-win-win situation. Examples are laser surgery, arthroscopy, lithotripsy, angioplasty, and recombinant DNA-based products. Because MRI increases cost over CT and other imaging methods, its growth has been somewhat enigmatic to date. However, ultra-low field strength MRI may change that and place it in the same category as the other breakthrough products.

CONCLUSION

The post-PPS competitive environment that has evolved in health care will continue to shape the industry well into the future. This chapter illustrates how the diffusion of technology is influenced by this environment. Each entity, payers, providers, and suppliers, will have an influence on how particular innovations are developed and used in health care settings. Thus, a symbiotic relationship develops in which each entity hopes to win. When all can win, the new technology will have a positive impact on the entire health care system.

ACKNOWLEDGMENTS

The authors thank Todd Storm of the University of Iowa for his competent research assistance.

17

The Impact of Multihospital System Affiliation on Decision-Making for Technology Adoption and Utilization

Paul E. Coakley, Jr.

The movement towards multihospital systems (MHS) has been consistent in recent years. This organizational technique is one approach hospitals have used to position themselves for dealing with an increasingly competitive market and a more businesslike industry approach. Multihospital systems have been defined as two or more hospitals owned, leased, sponsored, or managed by a single corporate entity (Alexander & Fennell, 1986). In contrast to independent, autonomous hospitals, these systems have grown from encompassing 24% of community hospitals and 32% of community hospital beds in 1975 to 44.3% and 43.9% of these categories, respectively, in 1986 (Provan, 1988).

Multihospital system affiliation has been studied from the perspective of its effect on the locus of decision-making authority. In the article cited above, Provan reviews both the theoretical literature on this issue and a series of empirical studies by himself and by Alexander and his colleagues. He states, based on this literature, that the type of system affiliation and its structure are important for understanding hospital decision-making autonomy. There has, however, been a relatively small amount of empirical literature on interorganizational dependence and decision-making autonomy. What has been done generally supports the position based on resource-dependence theory that there is a negative relationship between interorganizational dependence and decision-making autonomy. MHS affiliation is one of the most important forms of such dependence for a hospital (Provan, 1988).

While ultimate power is held by the parent organization in a multihospital organization, how that power is exercised through the delegation or concentration of decision-making authority is affected by conflicting motivations. Concentration permits coordination and control; delegation permits flexibility in reacting to local conditions. Multihospital systems can balance these opposing forces based on characteristics of the system and its member hospitals (Alexander & Fennell, 1986).

This chapter reviews the realities of affiliation with a multihospital system from the perspective of responsibility for the management of diagnostic and therapeutic services within an individual hospital that has become a member of such a system. The assessment is consistent with theorists who argue that organizations structure the decision-making process in such a way that its parameters tell people how they ought to choose (Huber & McDaniel, 1986; March & Simon, 1958; Simon, 1957, 1964).

The author's hospital formally affiliated with a multihospital system in 1987. Until then, it was autonomous for decision-making and financing although part of a loose association of hospitals. This association was based on each hospital being separately incorporated but owned by the same religious organization. There was cross-membership on the boards of directors of the individual hospitals and the benefits of group purchasing and the exchange of information among these hospitals.

With the affiliation into a multihospital system in 1987, a regional network of governing bodies was established. Each hospital must submit plans for major equipment purchases over $25,000 for corporate review and approval. Hospitals contribute to a central depository from which they can borrow for any approved purpose. However, corporate approval for purchases is independent of the source of funds to be used for the purchase.

The philosophy of this multihospital system is that health care is a local issue, and decision-making should be responsive to local needs. As a result, although corporate level controls financing, in actual practice it has never enforced a decision reversal. The orientation is towards providing a base of support and assistance to the individual hospitals in the system, not towards controlling their actions within the local setting. The management approach is not a "top down" dictation of technology policy, but a response to decisions requested from the the local level.

Given that contextual placement, the discussion that follows focuses in part on the realities of the current hospital environment as background to the potential benefits to be derived from multihospital system affiliation. It concludes with a review of the decision-making process relative to technology and on the differences in this for a hospital between independent status and system affiliation.

Three very important assumptions have been made as the basis for this discussion of the impact of system affiliation on hospital technology decision-making:

1. Health care costs will continue to escalate for the foreseeable future, creating the need for health service providers to become even more innovative in their adoption and utilization of technology in providing patient care.

2. Competition among facilities will intensify as external and internal factors reduce the demand for services from each health care facility.

3. The two conditions cited as assumptions above will create the need for the individual hospital to affiliate with a multihospital system or to enter into some other form of merger or consortia arrangement in order to survive into the 1990s.

Each of these three assumptions is supported by currently available data. Statistical analyses indicate the need for hospitals to affiliate to withstand the pressures brought to bear on them and to survive. The multihospital system appears to be the most beneficial vehicle to achieve this goal utilizing corporate control where necessary and maintaining a corporate philosophy of decision-making whenever possible at the individual health care facility level.

The health care industry continues to deal with these current pressures using a variety of different resources. In the author's opinion, the presence of the corporate chain of command within a multihospital system is an asset to the individual facility and to the community it serves. When it is established properly, its functioning focuses on the positive aspects of multihospital organizational structure.

Health care is considered to be, and rightly so, "big business." When the health care industry is looked at today, it is found to contain many of the aspects of private industry, i.e., profit margins, competition, effective and efficient use of resources, and the latest component, marketing. Particular reference is made to such components of the health care environment as market position, physician entrepreneurs, joint-venture opportunities, as well as mergers, acquisitions, and facilities that are closed or that fail.

First, we will analyze the current trends within the industry to identify the impact of the health care facility as a segment of a multihospital system. We will address the changes in corporate control and decision-making that are essential on a local level for the health care facility to survive and thrive. The health care industry today is experiencing a decline in the number of facilities providing patient care due to a reduction in the demand for the services offered.

The primary focus of patient care now is on the ambulatory (vertical) patient as opposed to the inpatient (horizontal patient). This trend has been developing over the past several years and has necessitated the individual facility making adjustments in the manner in which it provides patient care.

This reduction in the utilization of services has created an extremely competitive market that has intensified to the extent that rapid decision-making at the local level is paramount to success. The individual facility must be responsive to meeting this challenge in order to maintain and increase its patient population. However, being part of a larger organizational structure has many benefits, i.e., greater purchasing power for technology that is necessary for meeting the health care needs of today and greater leverage in negotiating contracts and in entering into various agreements, such as joint ventures, to strengthen its position.

Conversely, in many of the larger multihospital systems, decision-making often tends to be centrally located, and therefore the individual facility may face two primary dilemmas: (1) it is not able to respond rapidly to changes in the environment in which the facility must function, i.e., offering new services, obtaining new technology, and being able to meet or beat the competition that provides these services; (2) the allocation of funds for the procurement of such technology and new services also may be delayed because of the corporate bureaucracy that requires different levels of authorization or approval that take time to obtain.

If the multiinstitutional hospital system maintains a philosophy of supporting and strengthening the local facility with regard to localized decision-making, this enables the health care facility to respond to and compete from a much more favorable position. This more-favorable position affords the individual facility the opportunity to negotiate with the many varied populations with which it must come in contact. In addition, by making group procurements of the expensive technologies of today, significant savings may be realized with regard to obtaining MRI capability, lithotripsy, CT scanning, and many other high-cost technologies. Many facilities today are entering into joint-venture agreements with members of their attending staffs to defray all or part of the expense as well as the risk involved in obtaining these technologies. Having the support of a multihospital system provides even greater credibility with regard to support of such projects.

It is important here also to address the staffing requirements essential for operating newly acquired technology. Frequently, such staff are more inclined to work for larger organizations where they have not only the security and solidarity of the individual facility but also the opportunity to grow within the corporate chain as opportunities for advancement present themselves. Quite often the larger systems are much more able to provide benefits to their employees that are not available to smaller individual facilities. The larger multihospital systems frequently offer the opportunity to transfer within the corporate structure, which further enhances this benefit to an employee who may wish to relocate. The multihospital system also permits the reallocation of technology and other resources within the system so that the benefits of retaining this technology remain within the system.

An additional benefit derived from multihospital system affiliation is the research that quite often provides valuable information for the further enhancement of technology. Often financial grants and other sources of program funding tend to be directed towards the larger corporate facilities that typically can provide the resources to conduct the studies necessary for this data gathering and to share with the health care community the results of their work. The utilization of this funding also permits the acquisition of high-cost technology necessary for the research project.

The individual facility as a member of the multihospital system, therefore, should retain some degree of autonomy that would enable it to position itself properly in the local market. This aspect of belonging to the multihospital system but maintaining this local-level decision-making is critical to meeting the needs of the facility. It also permits the opportunity to deal with the physicians in the health care community in joint ventures previously mentioned, which can and does often further extend the resources of the facility. This joint venturing may take the shape of either two facilities joint venturing, or of this arrangement involving the facility and the physician-entrepreneur of today, who is at once both an ally and a competitor in the use of high technology. By realizing that the corporate control is such that these agreements may be reached on a local level, all parties may benefit.

The topic of costs must also be introduced and discussed to provide the reader with an overall picture of the advantages and disadvantages of multihospital systems. The purchasers of health care, i.e., the federal government, third-party insurance carriers, and the consumer, quite often can and will focus on the escalating costs of providing health care. There is a general feeling that technology is overutilized and therefore creates excessive costs to the purchaser of health care services. This is especially true where the duplication of services from one facility to another is present and therefore an overall increase in health care costs is realized. The multihospital system permits a broader perspective from which to examine the needs of the communities the respective individual hospitals serve as well as to view the procurement of the technology and the staffing to meet those needs.

At the corporate level the opportunity to obtain people with the expertise to coordinate the activities of the individual facilities is yet another benefit that can be realized. This expertise is helpful in consulting with each hospital in the system in the procurement of technology while at the same time obtaining substantial savings by multipurchase agreements with vendors. This practice may negate the relationship between the facility and the local vendor representative; however, the local vendor's role is also changing to that of providing informational services at the local level as an intermediary between the local facility and the corporate vendor.

Another factor that must be in evidence for the necessary decision-making to take place at the local level is effective communication within the system. Communication is essential to assure that the corporate resources are available when necessary and that guidance and direction are given where appropriate to the local facility. Corporate control and decision-making can have either a positive or a negative impact on the individual facility depending on how this is approached and practiced. It can and should be very beneficial when assisting with the analysis of new potential technologies. Often corporate decision-making requires the assistance and input of the local facility's expertise. This "marrying" of the local facility's resources and the support resources of the corporate level lends itself well to the success of decision-making in adopting new and upgraded technology.

In summary, the impact of the multihospital system on decision-making at the local level for adoption and utilization of technology results in lower costs of providing care to the patient/consumer. These reductions will be realized through the discounts obtained as a result of multifacility purchase, coordination with other facilities in technology procurement, and the introduction of state-of-the-art technology for both diagnostic and therapeutic testing. From the perspective of the author of this chapter, I see this as a definite benefit to all concerned, both providers and consumers. Corporate control is necessary and vital to assist the local facility in decision-making regarding technology procurement. The facility must appreciate and utilize this resource wisely.

This coordination of resources should also assist the individual facility in its response/reaction to competition at the local level. Multihospital systems typically are in a position to reallocate quickly resources to meet the needs of the community and the pressure from competition. If the individual facility that is part of the corporate system finds itself having to react to these pressures, the corporate network should be helpful here in assisting the facility in doing so. In a recent study by the Healthcare Financial Management Association of 1,400 hospitals, it was found that hospital profit margins are slipping and that the institutions are going to have increasing problems maintaining their facilities and the quality of service they offer. The number of hospital closures is expected to continue to increase and therefore the strength of the multiinstitutional hospital system continues to become more important.

The major advantages that this author sees as the benefit of multihospital system affiliation are coordination of efforts with other hospitals, group savings through preferred-provider arrangements, shared expertise, and the opportunity to locate another facility within the system that may be able to purchase equipment the hospital originally obtained but no longer derives sufficient use from to justify maintaining. When the hospital affiliated with the system, coordination of efforts and the increased strength of numbers in policy issues review relative to industry and governmental organizations were seen as decided pluses.

The impact of multihospital systems in corporate control and decision-making for adoption and utilization of technology is a rather significant one. This impact may be realized either positively or negatively depending on the corporate culture that is established. The effective use of the skills of a multihospital system will lead to the success desired. Improper use and lack of communication may only lead to failure. Multihospital systems must consider the alternatives and be prepared at all levels to make the proper moves to ensure success.

The availability of a corporate level for advice and consultation at any point in the hospital technology adoption and use decision-making process is a definite advantage. This opens a wider range of experience from within the system as well as information about the performance of specific providers and access to preferred providers. The corporate level offers the potential for a wider view of the market, sometimes resulting in the hospital deciding itself not to make a suggestion or to delay a purchase pending a more favorable price or product situation.

Having to go to the corporate level for review and approval above a set figure for purchases is a specific change from before to after affiliating with a multi-hospital system as far as technology decision-making is concerned. This requirement, though as indicated not one that has resulted in decision reversal, has impacted the decision-making process as it operates within the individual hospital. It has resulted in an increased orientation towards looking at alternatives and to lowering commitment to specific vendors. The awareness that there is another level of review outside the hospital itself probably has made staff members more sensitive to the need to review carefully and justify their requests. The overall process often provides and produces information that is invaluable to the decision-making process and strengthens it accordingly.

PART IV
IMPLICATIONS FOR TECHNOLOGY POLICY

18

Technology, Social Policy, and Social Change

Robert F. Rich and Noreen M. Sugrue

Public investment in science and technology is scarcely a novelty in the history of U.S. technological development. Indeed, the federal government was supporting scientific research as early as 1832 when the Treasury Department granted money to the Franklin Institute to study explosions of boilers on steamboats. At that time, however, the development of technology was not central for economic growth nor was it a centerpiece of our foreign policy.

Beginning with the Manhattan Project, which was organized for the narrow purpose of developing the atomic bomb, public investment in technological advancement has been critical for: (1) industrial recovery and economic growth in the Western world; (2) U.S. leadership in promoting the "technological revolution" as a way to combat communism; and (3) adoption of a public philosophy that promotes "technology for technology's sake."

One consequence of the choice of assigning such high priority to technological advancement—especially in the form of military and military-related projects—has been the neglect of pressing social and economic needs of society. The impacts of technological advance upon society and its environment became an issue of national importance in the late 1960s. Indeed, in an article published in 1970, Robert Gilpin points out that:

there is a growing belief that the United States must give greater attention to the formulation of a more explicit technological strategy designed to increase the social return of its immense investment in science and technology and to minimize its negative environmental effects. If this means, as it might, a slackening of economic growth, a cutback on military research, and a decline in commercially relevant innovations, the consequences for America's domestic politics, military posture, and international trade position would be significant. For this reason, the direction of America's technological strategy will become an increasingly important political issue. (Gilpin, 1970)

Gilpin is correct. This policy area has become an increasingly important political issue. Yet Gilpin's warning seems mild when compared with the convictions expressed by Gus Speth, Arthur Tamplin, and Thomas Cochran:

It is imperative that our society develop a capacity for saying no to technologies that are too risky and too demanding. We can no longer assume that each new innovation accompanied by financial backing should be permitted to proceed, even with regulation. (Speth, Tamplin & Cochran, 1976)

If as a society we have developed such a "capacity" to say *no* (because of the social risks involved) to the development of high technology that will stimulate the economy and advance our foreign policy goals, then we have come a long way since the Manhattan Project.

Historically, science and technology have been seen as means for achieving individual, organizational, and societal goals. In the 19th century, both Comte and Marx saw the development of technology as resulting in the emancipation of man; technology would allow men to be "free" and would give them more control over their lives. It would make the work environment more efficient and allow for more education and leisure time.

Since the industrial revolution, technology has been seen by many as the agent of social change (Mesthene, 1977). Technology has helped to foster steady incremental change throughout the social structure. Technology has been seen as improving the average quality of life, helping to foster economic growth, and helping to increase the economic and military power of this country.

As Dorothy Nelkin points out, the emphasis on science and technology as a means of achieving social and economic goals developed during the years following World War II (Nelkin, 1977). The importance of science to national peacetime policy became crucial after the Russians launched Sputnik in 1957 and the United States became committed to putting a man on the moon.

These developments led to increased federal funding of basic and scientific research and greater involvement of scientists in government. It has also led to a prolific literature in the field of science, technology, and public policy. This field is, however, generally unordered, and its scope remains poorly defined. This literature can be divided into several different types:

• The impacts of scientists in the formation of American public policy (e.g., Price, 1965; Gilpin, 1970; Sapolsky, 1974; Brooks, 1965.

- The existence of a scientific elite and its impact on society. The most interesting work in this area focuses on how scientific values permeate society as a whole (Ellul, 1964; Greenberg, 1967).
- A description of the R&D process.
- The making and implementing of science policy. This literature emphasizes the importance of administrative politics in controlling the growth of science and technology (Lanbright, 1976). This literature, building on the work of Price, also calls for greater accountability of the process of technological development (Price, 1965).
- The impact of international relations and military research on technology development and the international politics of national technology.

In this context, Gilpin points out:

A nation's choice of strategy reflects its social, economic, and security circumstances and objectives; therefore, the choice of strategy cannot be separated from the nation's broader domestic and foreign policies. Differing national strategies can be identified, but it must be noted that they are not exclusive strategies but rather characterize the major emphasis of a country's scientific and technological policies. (Gilpin, 1970)

This chapter builds on the literature focusing on science policy, values, social change, and their relationship to technology development. We argue that technology development should be viewed in the context of governmental and organizational decisions concerning investment in technology and innovation. Traditionally, there has been a calculus that has been adopted by most decision makers responsible for allocating financial and human resources to the development of research and technology. We label this calculus *the dominant model*. This model has been used to justify heavy investment in technology in the medical sciences and other high-tech areas. However, there is also an alternative model that is specified in this chapter; if one follows the assumptions imbedded in this model, a different decision calculus will emerge. We argue that this alternative model can and should be adopted in the field of medical technology as well as in areas of high technology in general.

DOMINANT MODEL OF DECISION-MAKING

Decisions about which research and development projects to fund and which not to fund have many social, political, and economic ramifications. There is little debate around the claim that technology, the end point of research and development projects, is "the single greatest source of economic development" (Volti, 1988, 16). There also is little controversy in claiming that there is a positive relationship between technological breakthroughs and economic development and competitiveness, and in some cases superiority (e.g., the United States prior to the late 1970s). Further, new knowledge and information obtained through any and all phases of research and development realign and restructure

Table 18.1
Assumptions and Decision Calculi of the Dominant Decision-Making Model for Research, Development, Technology, and Commercialization

- Research and development projects proceed in a linear fashion
- Research and development projects begin with basic research and continue, except in the rarest situations, through to commercialization
- In order to halt a research and development project prior to commercialization occurring, overwhelming and compelling evidence for stopping a project must be found
- Technology is evaluated as *a priori* good and desirable
- Technology is an outcome or end in itself
- The research team is not required to address the potential social, political, and economic consequences of its research
- Development of technology is positive, irrespective of how it may be applied
- When negative consequences of a research and development project occur, questions of responsibility and fault are assumed to be attributable to flaws in design or manufacturing
- The development of technology as technology enhances a society's competitive position and strengthens its economy
- A research and development project is evaluated on the basis of the technology produced

behaviors within the social, political, economic, legal, and ethical arenas (Volti, 1988).

Decisions about which research, development, technology, and commercialization projects to encourage and support historically have been driven by a model of decision-making that assumes all technologies and their applications are good. Further, the technology is thought to be beneficial on both individual and social planes. A summary of the assumptions of this decision-making model are found in Table 18.1. We now turn to a discussion of those assumptions.

Linearity

A research and development project from basic research through commercialization is conceived of as linear. That is, movement occurs as follows:

commercialization
technology
development of prototype
applied research
basic research

It can be thought of as a move up from one step to another, starting with basic research and culminating with commercialization. This is not to imply that information, data, and theories from other projects do not enter the process at various stages; in fact, just the opposite is the case. However, once you are at the stage of prototype development, you do not go back to the stage of applied research except in the most extreme circumstances (e.g., 75% of patients in a clinical drug trial die during the first month of a study). So if new information relevant to applied research is uncovered and the project already has begun to develop a prototype, in almost all situations there is not a return to the preceding stage.

Technology Is A Priori Good

The dominant model of decision-making is one that sees technology as, *a priori*, good, desirable, and beneficial. This is not to imply that there will be no negative costs or consequences associated with research, development, technology, and commercialization. In fact there will be, but the technology is assumed to be good. So for example, when *in vitro* fertilization was developed, it was assumed that any problems (e.g., social, legal, medical, or economic) associated with fertilization outside the womb would be worked out. In the final analysis, the ability to fertilize an egg outside a womb and transplant it into a womb was heralded as good prior to its application. It was thought to be good because capacity to perform a task was enhanced. In this sense the positive values of a technology and the positive values of its application are not distinguished. Rather, all technologies and their applications are necessary, needed, wanted, and valuable, prior to their implementation.

This commitment to technological development as good, *a priori*, leads to the following. Once basic research on a project has begun, it is assumed by all involved (e.g., scientists, funders, and policymakers) that the project will continue until a commercial product or technique is developed. In order for that not to occur, overwhelming evidence, evidence beyond a reasonable doubt if you will, against proceeding must be presented. Since the assumption is that the project is good and it will continue, those who want to stop the project must convince those responsible for the project that the work is not of value, is dangerous, or is otherwise harmful to persons or society. Because the quality and quantity of evidence required is so enormous, it is reasonable to claim that all but the fewest of projects continue on course.

Nonreflexivity

Another major assumption in this model is that members of the research team as well as other key decision-makers will not address social, economic, political, and ethical consequences of the data, information, and technology; that is, how data and products might be applied, how they might alter existing social arrangements, and a consideration of whether or not the project is worth the potential consequences are not part of the fundamental questions and issues confronted when deciding whether or not to proceed with a project. The assumption is that the application and its consequences are somebody else's arena and concern. The task before those involved in research and development is research and product development; potential or certain consequences of application are nonissues. When a negative consequence occurs (e.g., the crash of the Challenger), the research and development project and its goals are not questioned. Rather, the design or manufacturing process (e.g., how Morton Thiokol produced the O-rings) is investigated. Questions about the shuttle program and to what ends NASA is committing resources to this program are not entertained. Justification for the overall project is not required. Instead what is required is justification for how the findings and ideas that came out of the project were manufactured and applied.

Technology as an End

Within this decision-making frame, the development of technology is in itself an end. The evaluation of a research project is the very technology that is produced from it. What is occurring is research and development projects whose end is technology, and that technology is the outcome indicator of whether a research and development project has been successful. Questions of technology— for what reason, and why one project and technology over another—are not brought into the equation for deciding what to go ahead with.

Technology drives the research and development process. That is, as long as technology is produced, research and development projects get positively evaluated and are deemed successful. With successful research and development projects, it is easy to request and justify more research and development projects; if a team has a record of success, they are allowed to continue.

Technology and Economic Development

A final dimension to this decision-making model is one that sees technology as *the* engine for economic development, prosperity, and superiority. The more technology there is, the stronger the economy and the more likely a society is to have a high standard of living and international strength and power in business markets. Technology, or its lack, is *the* reason why some economic systems work and why some do not. If one examines where standard of living is high and where international economic power brokers look to for innovation, ideas, and leadership, it is those societies that see technology as, *a priori*, necessary and good.

This dominant model has driven and continues to drive the research and development process in the United States and other industrialized nations. In some ways it has served the U.S. economy very well (e.g., medical care, affordable housing, telecommunications). On the other hand, social, political, and economic consequences have been high (e.g., out-of-control inflationary health care costs, nuclear waste management, legal institutions that have no solutions to problems created by technology, for example, Baby Doe cases). To offer an analysis and critique of the dominant model without also offering an alternative model would be taking easy shots. In the following section we offer an alternative set of decision calculi for how to allocate resources and set priorities for research, development, technology, and commercialization. These, in some combination or another, have been infrequently employed. That is, these assumptions sometimes guide decisions, but all too rarely.

ALTERNATIVE MODEL OF DECISION-MAKING

This alternative model is not offered as a panacea. Rather, it is offered as a beginning point for examining new or alternative ways of deciding how to allocate and manage research and development. Research and development projects are a fundamental and necessary part of any industrialized economy. However, to assume, until otherwise proven that all research and development is good creates social institutions that contribute to and help sustain economic inflation and social problems.

Evolution and Reflexivity

The set of assumptions that drive this alternative model of decision-making are found in Table 18.2. These assumptions require persons responsible for decision-making with regards to research, development, technology, and commercialization to plan strategically and choose how resources are to be allocated and which projects are to be given priority based upon a comprehension of what likely costs and consequences will arise due to the project. The entire research and development process is set within the larger social arenas. That is, knowledge for knowledge's sake and technology for technology's sake, irrespective of impact on social institutions, is not an engine of the decision-making process. Instead, an engine for decision-making is the interaction and adaptation among the stages of the research and development process and the overall social structures. A consequence of this interaction and adaptation is that some of the work in and priorities of the research and development project and social institutions are altered and changed. So for example, as political, ethical, and environmental concerns about agriculturally related recombinant DNA research arose, the research and development process slowed up, stopped, and changed focus until more fundamental questions and issues were addressed (e.g., what are the environmental hazards, and is the research project worth those costs and risks?).

Table 18.2
Assumptions and Decision Calculi of the Alternative Decision-Making Model for Research, Development, Technology, and Commercialization

---

- Decisions, information, evaluations, and feedback are evolutionary and reflexive
- Technology as technology is neutral; its application is not
- It is incumbent upon members of the research team before the project begins, as well as during the duration of the project, to evaluate and judge the desirability and need for a research and development project in terms of likely economic, social, and political consequences of the knowledge and application generated from the project
- Decisions about research development, technology, and commercialization are made with careful attention to potential consequences
- Once a research and development project has begun, before the next phase or step is embarked upon, evaluations of opportunity costs as well as anticipated positive and negative consequences must occur
- Once a research and development project has begun, in order to continue it positive justification—reliable data and information—must be presented by the research team
- When there are negative social, economic, or political consequences as a result of a research and development project, evaluation of the project's overall premises must occur
- Technology is a means to an outcome
- The evaluation of research, development, technology, and commercialization occurs in terms of the overall goals and objectives that the project was to achieve; those goals and objectives are not to be the development of technology as technology

---

Evaluation of Consequences

Within this model the assumption is that technology as technology is neutral. However, neither the knowledge leading to technological development, nor its applications are neutral. The applications and uses carry social, political, economic, ethical, legal, and environmental consequences. Further, once knowledge has been disseminated, the ends to which it is applied cannot be controlled by the creator or anyone else for that matter; nor are we suggesting they should be. However, those involved in research and development need to be cognizant of and thoughtful about potential uses. Since there are numerous consequences, questions of why the research should be done, to what ends is it being done, and is it worth the likely risks, need to be asked and be considered as basic decisions about research and development projects are made. In this way, potential and likely outcomes are brought squarely into the decision-making process. Social, political, and environmental costs are as much a part of the decision-making process as is the availability of equipment and manpower.

These evaluations of likely costs should occur at all stages of a research and development project. The continuation of a project, regardless of costs and consequences, is due not to the innate momentum of having begun a research and development project but rather to the deliberate decision that the project, for a variety of reasons, ought to continue.

It also is important to indicate that even if there are minimal anticipated costs and consequences of a research and development project, positive justification for the project's continuation will occur at every stage. Persons directly involved in the research and development project need to give evidence that the project, as it is proceeding, is working towards its stated goals. Further, arguments for continued research allocations to the project are presented regularly. Since competition for scarce resources is stiff, each stage of every project needs to present sufficient cause for its opportunity costs.

When a significant negative impact occurs as a result of a research and development project, evaluations of the project itself must occur. A return to the Challenger example will illustrate this point. An analysis of the Challenger crash, under this model, requires in addition to investigating mechanical, design, and human mistakes a reexamination of why there is need of and support for the shuttle program. What are the purposes of the program? To what ends is the program aimed? Are the opportunity costs worth it? Are the ends to which the project is aimed reasonable for our society's current economic and political conditions? It is more than finding out what went wrong with the O-rings, the computers, or whatever. This model requires a rejustification of the entire research and development project. It further opens to debate and reevaluation the ends to which the project is aimed.

Technology as a Means to an End

This leads us to an important dimension of this alternative model: technology is a means. It is a means to achieving better health care, a cleaner environment, a more stable economy, a less-vulnerable defense system, and so on. Technology has no inherent value. Its value and worth reside in how effectively and efficiently it assists or enhances our abilities to reach socially acceptable goals and objectives. The value of a research and development project—was it successful?—is found in how well the project achieves its stated ends and how much of a contribution the knowledge and information from it make to other projects. These indicators are much more difficult to measure and evaluate. They require a less myopic view of research, development, technology, and commercialization, as well as a more detailed understanding of how the entire research and development process fits in to the larger social structure.

SUMMARY OF THE TWO DECISION-MAKING MODELS

While these two models share a basic concern, i.e., management of research and development projects, there is a fundamental difference between them. That difference is how decisions about the allocation and management of resources occur. The alternative model of decision-making looks at research and development as an evolutionary part of the overall social structure. As such, it interacts and adapts with the changing social environment. The dominant model sees research and development more independent of and detached from other social structures. Once a research and development project has begun, it takes on a life unto itself, and how it affects and alters other social arrangements is the concern and responsibility of persons other than those involved in the actual research and development.

We now turn to a discussion of the common themes found in the preceding chapters. Those themes coalesce around how research, development, technology, and commercialization have impacted health delivery in the United States.

COMMON THEMES

The authors of the preceding chapters offer analyses and critiques of technology proliferation within the health care arena. Although not framed in terms of decision-making models, these authors are fundamentally concerned with the consequences of technology—technology for what end? Why has medical technology expanded so dramatically and so quickly? What ends and purposes does medical technology serve? What have been the individual and organizational economic, political, ethical, and social consequences of biotechnology?

These questions, along with others, are basic to the alternative model of decision-making. They are, however, not part and parcel of the dominant model of decision-making. The authors raise a set of questions consistent with the alternative model. They tend to identify and describe problems, but not in terms of the underlying decision-making assumptions.

The problems highlighted in the previous chapters are a consequence of decisions about research, development, technology, and commercialization in health care being made within the dominant model.

Physician–Patient Relationships

One issue that is discussed throughout the chapters is the changed expectations of what medical care is. Fanton and Borenstein-Levy (Chap. 10) point out:

Modern medical technology has made a significant impact on the epidemiology and definition of disability, morbidity, and mortality. But in other respects, as well, the impact of its proliferation has been staggering. The expectations of patients or consumers have become more demanding; the job descriptions of the nurse, the doctor, and other health care practitioners have been altered; medical school curricula have been rewritten; and government and regulatory roles have been redefined. One cannot underestimate the impact of technology's proliferation.

The appearance of biotechnology has altered not only what patients expect of medical professionals but also how medicine is practiced. Moreover, it has produced a change in the numeric trends of indicators used to track the delivery and the quality of medical care. All of the authors concur with this point; and some, such as Riley and Brehm, point out that what the product is and how it is to be measured need to be defined in order to evaluate the changes in the delivery of health care due to technology. What has not accompanied the omnipresence of technology is a change or clarification in the definition of the desired outcomes of medical intervention. Brehm and Moulton, Rettig, and Maxwell and Sapolsky elaborate on the theme that availability of the latest technology is a proxy for quality of care. In addition, access to technology gets coded as access to the best possible medical care available. These situations are all reflective of decisions made with little, if any, attention paid to the potential consequences of research, development, technology, and commercialization, in other words, decisions made using the dominant model of decision-making.

That technology has changed how, where, to whom, and for what reasons medical interventions occur is not in dispute among these authors. Again, Fanton and Borenstein-Levy (Chap. 10) succinctly capture a concern common to the authors in this volume. They state ''[t]he questions become how best to research, develop, and utilize technology that will truly contribute to higher quality and economic efficiencies of health care, and at the same time eliminate technology that imposes costs not commensurate with delivered benefit.'' Finkelstein, Fanton and Borenstein-Levy, Mullner, Whiteis and Mullner, and Brehm and Mullner underscore that health care is given in ever-changing and complex social, economic, political, ethical, and medical arenas. They further point to the lack of research and theory about how the arenas reflect back upon each other and what the practical consequences of such interrelatedness are. The alternative decision-making model is one that forces members of the research team, as well as other key decision-makers (e.g., funders), to hinge their decisions about resource allocation on some of the very issues raised by the authors. So for example, how the development of HMOs has affected research and development with regard to biotechnology would be part and parcel of the alternative decision-making model. In addition, potential positive and negative ramifications would be considered, whereas with the dominant model of decision-making these issues are the concern and responsibility of others.

In the dominant model of decision-making, technology is the measurable outcome of how successful a research and development project has been. Under the alternative model, development and refinement of outcome measures is required before a project begins. What also is found within the alternative decision-making model is a feedback and reflexivity of data and information from all stages of the research and development process. Fanton and Borenstein-Levy, Krakauer, Brehm and Mullner, and Riley and Brehm discuss how evaluation and impact studies of biotechnology are designed and carried out. They are concerned with how data from these studies affect the development and application of technology, as well as how future resource allocation is impacted. The dominant model of decision-making does not address or in any way incorporate the concerns of these authors. The alternative model stresses the points that these authors raise as being fundamental to how resources for research, development, technology, and commercialization are allocated.

Consequences of Decisions Made Under the Dominant Model

The articles throughout this volume present the economic, political, social, and medical consequences of biotechnology. These consequences are a result of research, development, technology, and commercialization decisions made under the dominant model of decision-making. Many of the concerns and questions the authors raise are part of the decision calculi of the alternative model but not of the dominant model. So for example, Kimberly et al. raise the issue of what is the engine of technology, while Van Etten and Whiteis and Mullner, especially, are concerned with the question of technology for the sake of what ends. They, as do most of the authors throughout this volume, examine situations and consequences that are a result of the assumptions that more technology is better and that technology for the sake of technology is desirable.

Rosenberg, Brehm and Moulton, Brehm and Mullner, Maxwell and Sapolsky, Mullner, and Whiteis and Mullner reflect on the situations leading to and the consequences of linear fragmentary decision-making regarding delivery of service, utilization of technology, and reimbursement strategies for use of technology. While the dominant model of decision-making would not take these into account, the alternative model of decision-making would incorporate these issues, which are so fundamental to health care, into all stages of decision-making about research, development, technology, and commercialization. The tensions and choices among technological allocation, payment for use, and what is medically required and useful are enormous. This tension underscores the social, political, and economic residuals of technology for technology's sake.

Upon reflection, the chapters in this book offer solid empirical evidence that decisions made within the medical arena about commercialization of technology are made in a manner that does not require or support reflexivity and is fragmentary. These are decisions made under the dominant model described earlier in this chapter. The chapters underscore a need for rethinking the decision-making procedures and processes within the research, development, technology, and commercialization context. The question of to what ends and goals are decisions aimed needs to be a fundamental part of any decision-making processes concerned with resource allocation and management in research and development projects. These chapters underscore how necessary the assumptions and dimensions of our alternative decision-making model are if we are to understand decisions about and consequences of research, development, technology, and commercialization.

CONCLUSION

Research and development projects lead to new and improved technologies, regardless of which model of decision-making is employed. A key difference between the models is that for the dominant model, new or improved technologies always are sought after and are assumed, *a priori*, to be good. In the alternative model, new and improved technologies are outcomes, but only after debate, discussion, deliberation, and evaluation of the technologies and their possible impacts. In either case, however, the new or improved technologies alter, sometimes for better, sometimes for worse, the existing institutional arrangements. That is, the application of technology changes the way work and leisure activities are performed (e.g., stationary exercise bikes, personal computers, transistors, robots, food processors, psychotropic drugs, automated teller machines, among others). Social change is a necessary correlate of new or improved technologies. These changes may be as neutral or benign as people now being able to roast their own coffee beans at home, or as dramatic and far reaching, with debatable value, as the ability not to institutionalize chronic mentally ill patients because there are psychotropic drugs.

These changes that accompany technology also force members of society to reevaluate the rules, laws, and institutions that guide and maintain society. Many of these changes are so dramatic that existing social institutions cannot adapt and respond with enough flexibility to be effective. For example, our medical and legal institutions have not been able to adapt their rules, procedures, and ethics concerning parenthood when it involves a surrogate mother. The technology is available and workable; it has been tried and tested. However, whose child is it? Under what medical, social, legal, and ethical conditions ought surrogacy occur? What are the legal responsibilities of the medical personnel involved? These are but a few of the questions and issues produced by one procedure. Consensus on which questions to begin the discussion with, let alone agreement on answers, is nowhere in sight. Instead, we have a technology whose use is legally prohibited in some states, limited in others, and allowed to occur unencumbered in other states because we do not have existing social structures and experiences that we can incorporate with and adapt to this new method of becoming a parent. In fact, the technology has forced discussions of what is a parent, when does one become a parent, and under what conditions can parental responsibility be sold to another person? Numerous other examples in waste management, education, public health, business, and gene therapy, as well as other arenas, could be cited.

The induced social change forces reflection in two key areas. The first is concerned with how well social institutions are structured. Are they able to evolve and change when new ideas, thoughts, and behaviors are introduced? Can social institutions evolve along with the ideas and technologies developed by its people? If a society cannot adapt, what alternatives are available to its people? If the social institutions are not able to develop with changing ideas and technologies, where is the problem? That is, are the capacities of the institutions a limit of construction or are they due to the constructors' inability to do any better? If the legal system cannot bring into its sphere who is liable and responsible for protection of individual privacy even with the proliferation of easily accessible computerized data bases, is this because of a faultily designed legal system (i.e., is there a structural weakness or breaking point), or rather is the design the best people, at this point, can do? In other words, have the limits of man's abilities been reached in designing social institutions?

This leads us to the second area of concern. As technologies are developed and improved, are we stretching beyond the cognitive capabilities of people to deal with the consequences of technologies? Are people able to change and alter how they live, work, and recreate as quickly as the technologies are demanding? There is no doubt that man has the know-how to develop and implement new technologies; however, it is an open question whether or not man can adapt to those technologies. There are historical data that support man's ability to adapt and socially evolve given fundamental changes (e.g., the Industrial Revolution). There are, however, current situations that open to question man's ability to change with technologies and their consequences (e.g., acid rain, nuclear waste).

More work is needed not only in understanding how and why decisions about technology and resource allocation are made but also how individuals, organizations, and societies evolve with the technologies. For it is ultimately man's capability to develop and change entire social structures, given new technologies and their consequences, that is required for the maintenance and survival of our social structures.

Bibliography

Alexander, J. H., and Fennell, M. L. (1986). "Patterns of Decision Making in Multi-hospital Systems." *Journal of Health and Social Behavior* 27:14–27.

Altman, S. H., and Blendon, R., eds. (1979). *Medical Technology: The Culprit Behind Health Care Costs?* Hyattsville, Md: National Center for Health Services Research and Bureau of Health Planning. DHEW Publication no. PHS 79–3216.

American Hospital Association. (1974). *Capital Financing for Hospitals*. Chicago: American Hospital Association.

American Hospital Association. (1982). *Hospital Administration Terminology*. Chicago: American Hospital Publishing.

American Hospital Association. (1986). *Critical Choices: Capital Payments Under Medicare*. Washington, D.C.: American Hospital Association.

American Hospital Association. (1987). *Hospital Statistics*. Chicago: American Hospital Association.

American Hospital Association. (1988). *The State of the Nation's Access to Hospital Services*. Chicago: American Hospital Association.

Anderson, G. F., and Steinberg, E. P. (1984). "Hospital Readmissions in the Medicare Population," *New England Journal of Medicine* 311:1349–53.

Applebaum, E., and Granrose, C. S. (1986). "Hospital Employment Under Revised Medicare Payment Schedules," *Monthly Labor Review* 109, no. 8 (August): 37–45.

Arcidi, J. M.; Powelson, S. W.; King, S. B.; Douglas, J. S.; Jones, E. L.; Craver, J. M.; et al. (1988). "Trends in Invasive Treatment of Single-Vessel and Double-Vessel Coronary Disease." *Journal of Thoracic Cardiovascular Surgery* 95, no. 5 (May): 773–81.

Aries, N., and Kennedy, L. (1986). "The Health Labor Force: The Effects of Change." In *The Sociology of Health and Illness: Critical Perspectives*, P. Conrad and R. Kern, eds. pp. 196–206. 2d ed. New York: St. Martin's Press.

Arnould, R. J. (1987). "Issues in Financing Health Care: The Problem of Attaining an Efficient Capital Stock." Paper presented at the Public Policy Conference, *Health Care Policy: Where Is the Revolution Headed?* College of William and Mary, Williamsburg, Va: November 12–14.

Arnould, R. J., and DeBrock, L. M. (1986) "Competition and Market Failure in the Hospital Industry: A Review of the Evidence." *Medical Care Review* 43, no. 2 (Fall): 253–92.

Aronoff, B. L. (1986). "The State of the Art in General Surgery and Surgical Oncology." *Lasers in Surgery and Medicine* 6:376–82.

Averch, H., and Johnson, L. L. (1962). "Behavior of the Firm Under a Regulatory Constraint." *American Economic Review* 52 (December): 1052–69.

Baggish, M. S. (1986). "The State of the Art of Laser Surgery in Gynecology, 1985." *Lasers in Surgery and Medicine* 6:390–95.

Baim, D. S. (1988). "Interventional Cardiology—An Overview." *American Journal of Cardiology* 61, no. 14 (May 9): 1G–2G.

Baim, D. S., and Ignatius, E. J. (1988). "Use of Percutaneous Transluminal Coronary Angioplasty: Results of a Current Survey." *American Journal of Cardiology* 61, no. 14 (May 9): 3G–8G.

Barocci, T. A. (1981). *Non-Profit Hospitals: Their Structure, Human Resources and Economic Importance.* Boston, Mass.: Auburn House Publishing Company.

Berman, H. J.; Weeks, L. E.; and Kukla, S. F. (1986). *The Financial Management of Hospitals.* Ann Arbor, Mich.: Health Administration Press.

Bernstein, L. M.; Beaven, V. H.; Kimberley, J. R.; and Moch, M. K (1975). "Attributes of Innovation in Medical Technology and the Diffusion Process." In *The Diffusion of Medical Technology: Policy and Planning Perspectives*, G. Gordon and G. L. Fisher, eds. Cambridge, Mass.: Ballinger Publishing Co.

Blagg, C. (1977). "Cost of Dialysis and Transplantation." In *Strategy in Renal Failure*, E. Friedman, ed., 483–502. New York: John Wiley and Sons.

Bovbjerg, R.; Held, P.; and Pauley, M. (1982). "Procompetitive Health Insurance Proposals and their Implications for Medicare's End Stage Renal Disease Program." *Seminars in Nephrology* 2, no. 2 (June): 134–72.

Bradford, C.; Caldwell, G.; and Goldsmith, J. (1982). "The Hospital Capital Crisis: Issues for Trustees." *Harvard Business Review* (September–October): 1.

Brehm, H. P., and Coe, R. M. (1980). *Medical Care for the Aged: From Social Problem to Federal Program.* New York: Praeger.

Brentano, J., and Funck, J. L. (1985). "The Current Status and Future of the Artificial Kidney." *Artificial Organs* 9:119–26.

Brooks, H. (1965). "Scientific Concepts and Cultural Change." *Daedulus.* 93: 68–94.

Brown, J. B., and Saltman, R. B. (1985). "Health Capital Policy in the United States: A Strategic Perspective." *Inquiry* 22, no. 2 (Summer): 122–31.

Bruhn, J. G., and Philips, B. U. (1985). "The Influence of Technology on the Future of Allied Health Professionals." *Journal of Allied Health* (August): 289–95.

Bruton, P., and Waterman, J. (1985). "Capital Financing Demands New, Innovative Practices." *Healthcare Financial Management* (April): 38–45.

Bucci, V. A.; Reiss, J. B.; and Hall, N. C. (1985). "New Obstacles in the Path of

Marketing New Medical Devices; the Stream of Regulation." *Journal of Health Care Technology* 2, no. 2 (Fall): 81–96.

Bunker, J. P., and Schaffarzick, R. W. (1986). "Reimbursement Incentives for Hospital Care." *American Review of Public Health* 7: 391–409.

Califano, J. A. (1986). *America's Health Care Revolution*. New York: Random House, 3–10, 98, 101, 117, 160–67.

Chanard, J.; Brunois, J. P.; Melin, J. P.; Lavand, S.; and Toupance, O. (1985). "Long Term Results of Dialysis Therapy with a Highly Permeable Membrane," *Artificial Organs* 6:261–66.

Chaussy, C.; Brendel, W.; and Schmiedt, E. (1980). "Extracorporeally Induced Destruction of Kidney Stones by Shock Waves." *The Lancet* 8207 (December 13) (1980–2):1265–68.

Chaussy, C.; Schmiedt, E.; Jocham, D.; Brendel, W.; Forssman, B.; and Walther, V. (1982). "First Clinical Experience with Extracoreally Induced Destruction of Kidney Stones by Shock Waves." *Journal of Urology* 127, no. 3 (March): 417–20.

Coddington, D. C.; Palmquist, L. E.; and Trollinger, W. V. (1985). "Strategies for Survival in the Hospital Industry." *Harvard Business Review* 63 (May–June): 129–39.

Cohodes, D. R., and Kinkead, B. M. (1984). *Hospital Capital Formation*. Baltimore: Johns Hopkins University Press.

Committee on Technology and Health Care, National Research Council. (1979). *Medical Technology and the Health Care System: A Study of the Diffusion of Equipment-Embodied Technology*. Washington, D.C.: National Academy of Sciences.

CommonHealth. (1983). "Understanding Massachusetts' New Hospital Law." *Staying Alive!* (February).

Council on Scientific Affairs. (1986). "Lasers in Medicine and Surgery." *Journal of the American Medical Association* 256, no. 7 (August 15): 900–907.

Cowley, M. J.; Vetrovec, G. W.; DiSciascio, G.; Lewis, S. A.; Hirsh, P. D.; and Wolfgang, T. C. (1985). "Coronary Angioplasty of Multiple Vessels: Short-Term Outcome and Long-Term Results." *Circulation* 72, no. 6 (December): 1314–20.

Cox, D. R., and Oakes, D. (1984). *Analysis of Survival Data*. London: Chapman and Hall.

Crawford, M., and Fottler, M. D. (1985). "The Impact of Diagnosis Related Groups and Prospective Pricing Systems on Health Care Management." *Health Care Management Review* 10, no. 4: 73–84.

Dalton, M. "Conflict between Staff and Line Managerial Officers." In *A Sociological Reader on Complex Organizations*, Etzioni, A., ed., 226–74, 2d ed. New York: Holt, Reinhart & Winston, Inc.

Dans, P. E.; Weiner, J. P.; and Otter, S. E. (1985). "Peer Review Organizations." *New England Journal of Medicine* 313:1131–37.

Davis, A. B. (1981). *Medicine and Its Technology*. Westport, Conn.: Greenwood Press.

Davis, C. K. (1982). "Proposed Prospective Reimbursement Rates for the End Stage Renal Disease Program." Testimony before the U.S. Senate Committee on Finance, Subcommittee on Health (March 15).

Deane, N., and Bemis, J. (1983). "Multiple Use of Hemodialyzers." In *Replacement of Renal Function by Dialysis*, ed. W. Drukker. Boston: Martinus Nijhoff Publishers.

DeBakey, M. E., (1976). Cardiac Surgeon, speaking at *National Leadership Conference on America's Health Policy* (April 29).

Demkovich, L. E. (1980). "Even When It Is Giving Out Money, HEW Can't Escape Controversy." *National Journal* 12, no. 15 (April 12): 604–6.

Department of Health and Human Services (1984). *Report to the President and Congress on the Status of Health Personnel in the United States*. Vol. 1. DHHS Publication no. HRS-P-OD 84–4 (May).

Detre, K.; Holubkov, R.; Kelsey, S.; Cowley, M.; Kent, K.; Williams, D.; et al. (1988). "Percutaneous Transluminal Coronary Angioplasty in 1985–1986 and 1977–1981." *The New England Journal of Medicine* 318, no. 5 (February 4): 265–70.

Drukker, W. (1983a). "Peritoneal Dialysis: A Historical Review." In *Replacement of Renal Function by Dialysis*, ed. W. Drukker. Boston: Martinus Nijhoff Publishers.

Drukker, W. (1983b). "Hemodialysis: A Historical Review," In *Replacement of Renal Function by Dialysis,* ed. W. Drukker. Boston: Martinus Nijhoff Publishers.

Easterbrook, G. (1987). "The Revolution in Medicine." *Newsweek* (January 26): 40–74.

Eddy, D. M. (1980). *Screening for Cancer: Theory, Analysis and Design*. Englewood Cliffs, N.J.: Prentice-Hall.

Egdahl, R. H. (1987). "The Pressure on Physicians to Economize: The Impact of Managed Care Programs on Medical Practice." Conference keynote address: *Health Technology Adoption in a DRG Age*, Center for Technology and Policy, Boston University (September).

Egdahl, R. H., and Walsh, D. C., eds. (1985). *Health Cost Management and Medical Practice Patterns*. Cambridge, Mass.: Ballinger Publishing Co.

Eggers, P. W. (1984). "Trends in Medicare Reimbursement for End-Stage Renal Disease: 1974–1979." *Health Care Financing Review* 6:31–38.

Eggers, P. W.; Connerton, R.; and McMullan, M. (1984). "The Medicare Experience with End Stage Renal Disease: Trends in Incidence, Prevalence, and Survival." *Health Care Financing Review* 5, no. 3 (Spring): 69–87.

Ellul, J. (1964). *The Technological Society*. London: Jonathon Casey.

Elrod, J. L., and Wilkinson, J. A. (1985). *Hospital Project Financing and Refinancing Under Prospective Payment*. Chicago: American Hospital Association.

Enthoven, A. C., and Noll, R. G. (1984). "Prospective Payment: Will It Solve Medicare's Financial Problem?" *Issues in Science and Technology* 1: 101–16.

Ermann, D., and Gabel, J. (1984). "Multihospital Systems: Issues and Empirical Findings." *Health Affairs* 3, no. 1 (Spring): 50–64.

Evens, R. G.; Jost, R. G.; and Evens, R. G., Jr. (1985). "Economics and Utilization Analysis of Magnetic Resonance Imaging Units in the United States in 1985." *American Journal of Radiology* 145 (August): 393–98.

Federal Register. (1986). (May 13): 17540.

Federal Register. (1983). Vol. 48, no. 92 (May 11): 21254.

Fein, Rashi. (1986). *Medical Care, Medical Costs*. Cambridge, Mass.: Harvard University Press, 82, 86, 87.

Feldstein, M. (1981). "The Rapid Rise of Health Costs." In *Health Costs and Health Insurance*. Cambridge, Mass.: Harvard University Press.

Feldstein, P. J. (1966). "An Analysis of Alternative Reimbursement Plans." In *Reimbursement Incentives of Hospital and Medical Care*, U.S. Department of Health,

Education, and Welfare, Social Security Administration Research Report no. 26, 17–38.

Feldstein, P. J. (1983). *Health Care Economics*. 2d ed. New York: John Wiley & Sons, 213–23, 292–93.

Food and Drug Administration, Center for Devices and Radiological Health, Office of Device Evaluation. (1986). *Annual Report*, Fiscal Year.

Fries, J. F. (1984). "The Chronic Diseases Data Bank: First Principles to Future Directions." *Journal of Medical Philosophy* 9:161–80.

Geyer, O., and Lazar, M. (1986). "Laser Therapy of Eye Diseases." *Lasers in Surgery and Medicine* 6:423–26.

Gilpin, R. (1970). "Technological Strategies and National Purpose," *Science* Vol. 169, no. 3944 (July 31): 441–48.

Glenn, K. (1984). *Capital Financing in the 1980s: An Essential Guide for Hospital Management*. Washington, D.C.: McGraw-Hill.

Golden, P. M.; Wilson, R. W.; and Kavet, J. (1984). *Health, United States, 1984*. DHHS Publication no. PHS 84–1232. Public Health Service. Washington, D.C.: U.S. Government Printing Office.

Goldfarb, M. G.; Hornbrook, M. C.; Kelly, J. V.; and Monheit, A. C. (1980). "Health Care Expenditures." *Health, United States, 1980*, DHHS Publication no. PHS 81–1232. Public Health Service. Washington, D.C.: U.S. Government Printing Office, 101–16.

Gordon, G.; MacEachron, A. E.; and Fisher, G. L. (1975). "Perspectives on Diffusion Research." In *The Diffusion of Medical Technology: Policy and Planning Perspectives*, G. Gordon and G. L. Fisher, eds. Cambridge, Mass.: Ballinger.

Graham, M. B. W., and Rosenthal, S. R. (1986). *Institutional Aspects of Process Procurement for Flexible Machining Systems*. Manufacturing Roundtable, Boston University (September).

Greenberg, D. S. (1967). *The Politics of Pure Science*. New York: American Library.

Greer, A. L. (forthcoming). "Rationing Medical Technology: Hospital Decision-Making in the United States and England." *International Journal of Technology Assessment in Health Care*.

Guterman, S., and Dobson, A. (1986). "Impact of Medicare Prospective Payment System for Hospitals." *Health Care Financing Review* 7, no. 3 (Spring): 97–114.

Haik, K. G.; Terrell, W. L.; and Haik, G. M. (1987). "Lasers in Ophthalmology Today." *Journal of the Louisiana State Medical Society* 139, no. 9 (September): 32–37.

Hall, R. H. (1972). *Organizations: Structure and Process*. 1st ed. Englewood Cliffs, N.J.: Prentice-Hall.

Hall, R. H. (1982). *Organizations: Structure and Process*. 3d ed. Englewood Cliffs, N.J.: Prentice-Hall.

Halper, T. (1986). "End Stage Renal Failure and the Aged in the United Kingdom." *International Journal of Technology Assessment in Health Care* 1, no. 1 (January): 41–53.

Hardin, Garret. (1968). "The Tragedy of the Commons." *Science* 162, no. 3859: 1243–48.

Harrell, F. (1983). "The PHGLM Procedure." In *SUGI Supplemental Library User's Guide*. 1983 ed. Cary, N.C.: SAS Institute.

Hartzler, G. O.; Rutherford, B. D.; McConahay, D. R.; Johnson, W. L.; and Giorgi,

L. V. (1988). "High Risk Percutaneous Transluminal Coronary Angioplasty." *American Journal of Cardiology* 61, no. 14: 33G–37G.

Health Care Financing Administration. (1983). "Medicare program; prospective payment for Medicare inpatient services." *Federal Register* (September 1): 48:39752–890.

Health Care Financing Administration. (1984). End-Stage Renal Disease Program Highlights.

Henderson, J. A. (1987). "Cost Containment, Hospital Competition Aren't Limiting Surgery Center Expansion." *Modern Healthcare* 17, no. 12:148–54.

Hernandez, M. D., and Howie, C. G. (1979). "Capital Financing by Multihospital Systems." In *Multihospital Arrangements: Public Policy Implications*, Y. S. Mason, ed., 37–47. Chicago: American Hospital Association.

Hertzberg, R. (1986). "A Short History of Ophthalmic Laser." *Australian and New Zealand Journal of Ophthalmology* 14:387–88.

Herzlinger, R., and Krasker, W. (1987). "Who Profits from Nonprofits?" *Harvard Business Review* (January–February).

Hiatt, H. H. (1975). "Protecting the Medical Commons: Who Is Responsible." *New England Journal of Medicine* 293, no. 5: 235–41.

Hillman, A. L., and Schwartz, J. S. (1985). "The Adoption and Diffusion of CT and MRI in the United States: A Comparative Analysis." *Medical Care* 23, no. 11 (November): 1283–94.

Hoenitch, N., and Kerr, D. (1983). "Dialyzers." In *Replacement of Renal Function by Dialysis*, W. Drukker, ed. Boston: Martinus Nijhoff Publishers.

Holmes, D. R. Jr.; Reeder, G. S.; and Vlietstra, R. E. (1988). "Role of Percutaneous Transluminal Coronary Angioplasty in Multivessel Disease." *American Journal of Cardiology* 61, no. 14 (May 9): 9G–14G.

Holoweiko, M. (1983). "How Doctors Kicked Out a Hospital Board." *Medical Economics* 60, part 14 (July): 92–98, 102.

Huber, G., and McDaniel, R. (1986). "The Decision-Making Paradigm of Organizational Design." *Management Science* 32:572–89.

Iglehart, J. K. (1986). "Health Policy Report: Early Experience with Prospective Payment." *New England Journal of Medicine* 314, no. 22 (May): 29, 1460–64.

Jacobs, D. (1974). "Dependency and Vulnerability: An Exchange Approach to the Control of Organizations." *Administrative Science Quarterly* 19, no. 1 (March): 45–59.

Joffe, S. N., and Schroder, T. (1987). "Lasers in General Surgery." *Advances in Surgery* 20:125–54.

Kahl, A., and Clark, D. E. (1986). "Employment in Health Services: Long-term Trends and Projections." *Monthly Labor Review* 109, no. 8 (August): 17–36.

Kinkead, B. M. (1984). "Medicare Payment and Hospital Capital: The Evolution of Policy." *Health Affairs* 3, no. 3 (Fall): 49–74.

Kotelchuck, R. (1986). "In the Grip of PPS: How Prospective Payment is Transforming Hospital Care." *Health/PAC Bulletin* 17, no. 1 (November): 7–10.

Kraebber, D., and Torres, S. (1988). "Extracorporeal Shock Wave Lithotripsy: Review of the First 100 Cases at the Kidney Stone Center of Southeast Georgia." *Southern Medical Journal* 81, no. 1 (January): 48–51.

Krakauer, H. (1986). "Assessment of Alternative Technologies for the Treatment of End-Stage Renal Disease." *Israel Journal of Medical Sciences* 22:245–59.

Krakauer, H.; Grauman, J. S.; McMullan, M. R.; and Creede, C. C. (1983). "The

Recent U.S. Experience in the Treatment of End-Stage Renal Disease by Dialysis and Transplantation." *New England Journal of Medicine* 308:1558–61.

Kusserow, R. P. (1982). Testimony before the Subcommittee of the Committee on Government Operations. U.S. House of Representatives (February 23–24); 7–17.

Laffey, W. J., and Lappen, S. (1976). "Tax-Exempt Hospital Financing: Revenue Bonds." *Health Care Management Review* 1, no. 4 (Fall): 19–30.

Lanbright, W. H. (1976). *Governing Science and Technology.* New York: Oxford University Press.

Langwell, K. M., and Moore, S. F. (1982). *A Synthesis of the Research on Competition in the Financing and Delivery of Health Services.* DHHS Publication no. PHS 83–3327. National Center for Health Services Research, U.S. Public Health Service.

Leonard-Barton, D., and Deschamps, I. (1989). "Managerial Influence in the Implementation of New Technology." *Management Science* (forthcoming).

Levey, S., and Loomba, N. P. (1984). *Health Care Administration: A Managerial Perspective.* 2d ed. Philadelphia: J. B. Lippincott Co.

Lewin & Associates, Inc. (1987). *Medical Supplies and Phamaceuticals: A Summary of Hospital and Manufacturer Interview and Data Analysis Concerning the Impact of Medicare's Prospective Payment System.* Prepared for the Prospective Payment Assessment Commission, Contract No. T–33731757. Washington, D.C. (April).

Litvack, F.; Grundfest, W. S.; Papaioannou, T.; Mahr, F. W.; Jakubowski, A. T.; and Forrester, J. S. (1988). "Role of Laser and Thermal Ablation Devices in the Treatment of Vascular Diseases." *American Journal of Cardiology* 61, no. 14 (May 9): 81G–86G.

Lowrie, E. G., and Hampers, C. L. (1981). "The Success of Medicare's End Stage Renal Disease Program." *New England Journal of Medicine* 305, no. 8 (August 20): 434–38.

Lowrie, E. G., and Hampers, C. L. (1984). "Medicare's End-Stage Renal Disease Program: Historical and Policy Considerations." In *Controversies in Nephrology and Hypertension.* R. G. Narins, ed., 8. New York: Churchill Livingstone Inc.

"Magnetic Resonance Imaging." (1988). Editorial, *American Family Physician* 37, no. 6 (June): 91–92.

Maloney, T. W., and Rogers, D. E. (1979). "Medical Technology—A Different View of the Contentious Debate Over Costs." *New England Journal of Medicine* 301, no. 26 (December): 1413–19.

Marberger, M.; Turk, C.; and Steinkogler, I. (1988). "Painless Prezoelectric Extracorporeal Lithotripsy." *Journal of Urology* 139, no. 4 (April): 695–99.

March, J., and Simon, H. (1958). *Organizations.* New York: John Wiley & Sons.

Marcson, S. (1962). "Decision Making in a University Physics Department." *American Behavioral Scientist* 6, no. 4 (December): 37–39.

Massachusetts Hospital Association. "The Medicare Prospective Payment System: Management and Policy Implications." *Management and Policy Brief* 2, no. 2.

Maxwell, J. H. (1986). "The Iron Lung: Halfway Technology or Necessary Step." *Milbank Memorial Fund Quarterly, Health and Society* 64, no. 1: 3–29.

McNeil, B. J., and Cravalho, E. G. (1982). *Critical Issues in Medical Technology.* Boston: Auburn House Publishing Company, 51–91.

Mechanic, D. (1985). "Cost Containment and the Quality of Medical Care: Rationing

Strategies in an Era of Constrained Resources." *Milbank Memorial Fund Quarterly, Health and Society* 63, no. 3: 453–75.

Mesthene, E. G. (1977). "The Role of Technology in Society." In *Technology and Man's Future*, A. Teich, ed. New York: St. Martin's Press.

Metz, M. (1983). "Trends in Sources of Capital in the Hospital Industry." In *Report of the American Hospital Association Special Committee on Equity of Payment for Not-For-Profit and Investor-Owned Hospitals*, Appendix D. Chicago: American Hospital Association (May).

Miller-Catchpole, R. (1988a). "Diagnostic and Therapeutic Technology (DATTA) Ureteral Stone Management: The Use of Ureteroscopy with Extracorporeal Shock Wave Lithotripsy or Ultrasonic Lithotripsy." *Journal of the American Medical Association* 259, no. 9 (March 4): 1382–84.

Miller-Catchpole, R. (1988b). "Diagnostic and Therapeutic Technology (DATTA) Ureteral Stone Management: II. Ureteroscopy and Ultrasonic Lithotripsy." *Journal of the American Medical Association* 259, no. 10 (March 11): 1557–59.

Morris, D. C. (1988). "Coronary Angioplasty: A Cardiologist's Perspective." *Journal of Thoracic Cardiovascular Surgery* 95, no. 5 (May): 758–60.

Morse, E. V.; Gordon, G.; and Moch, M. (1974). "Hospital Costs and Quality of Care: An Organizational Perspective." *Milbank Memorial Fund Quarterly, Health and Society* 52, no. 3: 315–46.

Moscovice, I. (1988). "Health Care Professionals." In *Introduction to Health Services*, S. J. Williams and P. R. Torrens, eds., 308–34. New York: John Wiley & Sons.

Moss, N. P. (1988). Personal Communication with Neil P. Moss, President, National Council of Health Facilities Financing Authorities (January).

National Center for Health Statistics. 1980–1985. *Utilization of Short-Stay Hospitals*. U.S. Hospitals Annual Survey, Hospital Discharge Survey, series 13, by year from 1980 to 1985.

National Committee for Quality Health Care. (1987). *Medical Technology in the Competitive Market*. White paper of the Task Force on Medical Technology (February).

National Health Lawyer's Association. (1982). "Capital Financings and Refinancings for Health Care Facilities." Paper presented on January 20–22, Washington, D.C.

Nelkin, D. (1977). "Technology and Public Policy." In *Science, Technology, and Society: A Cross-Disciplinary Perspective*, I. Spiegel-Rosing and D. de Solla Price, eds. Beverly Hills, Calif.: Sage, 393–441.

Neuhauser, D. (1983). "The Future of Technology and Manpower in Medical Care." In *Health Care Financial Management in the 1980s: Time of Transition*, J. B. Silvers, W. N. Zelman, and C. N. Kahn, ed. Ann Arbor, Michigan, and Washington, D.C.: AUPHA Press.

Newhouse, J. P. (1978). "The Structure of Insurance and the Erosion of Competition in the Medical Marketplace." In *Competition in the Health Care Sector: Past, Present and Future*, W. Greenberg, ed. Germantown, Md: Aspen Systems Corporation.

Office of Technology Assessment. U.S. Congress. (1985). *Medicare's Prospective Payment System: Strategies for Evaluating Cost, Quality, and Medical Technology*. OTA-H-262, Washington, D.C.: U.S. Government Printing Office (October). Republished by Springer Publishing Co., New York, 1986.

Page, J. (1982). "A Case of Technocide." *Science* 3, no. 9 (November): 93–94.

Pozen, M. W.; Lerner, D. J.; D'Agostino, R. B.; Strauss, H. W.; and Gertman, P. M. (1984). "Cardiac Nuclear Imaging: Adoption of an Evolving Technology." *Medical Care* 22, no. 4 (April): 343–48.

Price, D. K. (1965). *The Scientific Estate*. Cambridge, Mass.: Harvard University Press.

Prospective Payment Assessment Commission. (1986). *Technical Appendixes to the Report and Recommendations to the Secretary, U.S. Department of Health and Human Services*. Washington, D.C.: U.S. Government Printing Office (April 1).

Prospective Payment Assessment Commission. (1987). *Technical Appendixes to the Report and Recommendations to the Secretary, U.S. Department of Health and Human Services*. Washington, D.C.: U.S. Government Printing Office (April 1).

Prottas, J., and Sapolsky, H. M. (1980). "Retreat to Regulation: Administration of the End Stage Renal Disease Program." Unpublished paper, University Health Policy Consortium. Cambridge, Mass.: MIT.

Prottas, J., and Sapolsky, H. M. (1981). "Administrative Problems in the End Stage Renal Disease Program." Unpublished paper. University Health Policy Consortium. Cambridge, Mass.: MIT.

Prottas, J.; Segal, M.; and Sapolsky, H. M. (1983). "Cross-National Differences in Dialysis Rates." *Health Care Financing Review* 4, no. 3 (March): 91–103.

Provan, K. (1988). "Organizational and Decision Unit Characteristics and Board Influence in Independent versus Multihospital System-Affiliated Hospitals." *Journal of Health and Social Behavior* 29 (September): 239–52.

Public Health Service. *Health, United States, 1987*. (1988) DHHS Publication no. (PHS)88–1232. Table 63: *Discharges, Days of Care, and Average Length of Stay in Nonfederal Short-Stay Hospitals, According to Selected Characteristics: United States, 1980–86*. Washington, D.C.: U.S. Government Printing Office.

Raffel, M. W. (1984). *The U.S. Health System: Origins and Functions*. New York: John Wiley & Sons.

Reeder, G. S.; Krisham, I.; Nobrega, F. T.; Naessens, J.; Kelly, M.; Christianson, J. B.; and McAfee, M. K. (1984). "Is Percutaneous Coronary Angioplasty Less Expensive than Bypass Surgery?" *New England Journal of Medicine* 311, no. 18 (November 1): 1157–62.

Reilly, N., and Torosian, L. (1988). "The New Wave Lithotripsy: Implications for Nursing." *RN* 51, no. 3: 44–48.

Rettig, R. (1980). "The Politics of Health Cost Containment: End Stage Renal Disease." *Bulletin of the New York Academy of Medicine* 56:115–38.

Rettig, R. (1982). "The Federal Government and Social Planning for End Stage Renal Disease: Past, Present, and Future." *Seminars in Nephrology* 2, no. 2 (June): 111–33.

Rettig, R. (1986). "Treatment of End Stage Renal Disease: Some Policy Lessons from the Seattle Experience." *Dialysis and Transplantation* 15, no. 1 (January): 12–13.

Rettig, R., and Marks, E. (1980). "Implementing the End Stage Renal Disease Program of Medicare." Report to the Health Care Financing Administration. Washington, D.C.: Office of Research, Demonstration and Statistics/U.S. Department of Health and Human Services.

Rice, D. P., and Feldman, J. J. (1983). "Living Longer in the United States: Demographic Changes and Health Needs of the Elderly." *Milbank Memorial Fund Quarterly, Health and Society* 61, no. 3: 362–96.

Riley, G., and Lubitz, J. (1985). "Outcomes of Surgery among the Medicare Aged: Surgical Volume and Mortality." *Health Care Financing Review* 7:37–48.

Roberts, E. (1982). "The Development of Medical Technologies." In *Critical Issues in Medical Technology*, B. J. McNeil and E. G. Cravalho, eds. Boston: Auburn House Publishing Company.

Roberts, E. B.; Levy, R. I.; Finkelstein, S. N.; Moskowitz, J.; and Sondik, E. J. (1981). *Biomedical Innovation*. Cambridge, Mass.: Massachusetts Institute of Technology Press.

Rock, R. C. (1985). "Assuring Quality of Care under DRG-Based Prospective Payment." *Medical Decision Making* 5:31–34.

Rogers, E. M. (1983). *Diffusion of Innovations*. New York: The Free Press.

Romeo, A. (1984). "Health Case Study 32: The Hemodialysis Equipment and Disposables Industry." Washington, D.C.: Office of Technology Assessment.

Rosenberg, N. (1976). *Perspectives on Technology*. Cambridge University Press, 9–31.

Rosengren, W. R. (1980). *Sociology of Medicine: Diversity, Conflict, and Change*. New York: Harper & Row, 191–93.

Rosenstein, A. H. (1986). "Hospital Closure or Survival: Formula for Success." *Health Care Management Review* 11, no. 3: 29–35.

Rosenthal, S. R. (1984). "Progress Toward the Factory of the Future." *Journal of Operations Management* 4, no. 3 (May): 203–29.

Rubin, R. J. (1984). "Epidemiology of End Stage Renal Disease and Implications for Public Policy." *Public Health Reports* 99: 492–98.

Rubin, R. J.; Moran, D. W.; Jones, K. S.; and Hackbarth, M. A. (1988). *Critical Condition: America's Health Care in Jeopardy*. Report to the National Committee for Quality Health Care. Washington, D.C.: Lewin/ICF, Health and Sciences Research, Inc.

Russell, L. B. (1979). *Technology and Hospitals: Medical Advances and Their Diffusion*. Washington, D.C.: Brookings Institution.

Sadler, J. (1981). "ESRD Program Operations and Management." Hearings before the Subcommittee on Health, Committee on Finance, U.S. Senate, 155.

Salkever, D. S., and Bice, T. W. (1976). "The Impact of Certificate-of-Need Controls on Hospital Investment." *Milbank Memorial Fund Quarterly* 54, no. 2; (Spring): 185–214.

Sapolsky, H. M. (1974). *The Polaris Development: Bureaucratic and Programmatic Success in Government*. Cambridge, Mass.: Harvard University Press.

Sapolsky, H. M.; Aisenberg, J.; and Morone, J. (1987). "The Call to Rome and Other Obstacles to State-Level Innovation." *Public Administration Review* (March).

Schwartz, W. (1987). "The Inevitable Failure of Cost-Containment Strategies." *Journal of American Medicine* 257, no. 2 (January 9) 220–21.

Shapleigh, T. (1985). "The Use of Data for Health Cost Management at New England Medical Center: Case Management, Product Pricing, and Concurrent Reporting of Resource Utilization." In *Health Cost Management and Medical Practice Patterns*. R. H. Egdahl and D. C. Walsh, eds. Cambridge, Mass.: Ballinger Publishing Company.

Shaw, S. H. (1985). "The Compelling Issue of Access to Capital." *Business and Health* (January/February): 17–20.

Sidel, V. W., and Sidel, R. (1983). "Health Care and Medical Care in the United States." In *A Healthy State*. Pantheon Books: New York, 3–112.

Siegel, D. M. (1987). "The High Cost of Medical Technology: Getting at the Heart of the Matter." *Medical Care* 25, no. 10 (October): 979–87.

Simon, H. (1957). *Administrative Behavior*. 2d ed. New York: Macmillan.

Simon, H. (1964). "On the Concept of Organizational Goal." *Administrative Science Quarterly* 9:1–22.

Sloan, F. A. (1981). "Regulation and the Rising Cost of Hospital Care." *Review of Economics and Statistics* 58, no. 4 (Fall): 479–87.

Sorian, R. (1987). Special Report. *Medicine and Health* (December 28).

Speck, B.; Bortin, M. M.; Champlin, R.; Goldman, J. M.; Herzig, R. H.; McGlave, P. B.; Messner, H. A.; Weiner, R. S.; and Rimm, A. A. (1984). "Allogeneic Bone Marrow Transplantation for Chronic Myelogenous Leukemia." *Lancet* 1, no. 8378:665–68.

Speth, G.; Tamplin, A; and Cochran, T. (1976). *Nuclear Moratorium*. Washington, D.C.: Environmental Action Foundation.

Stason, W., and Barnes, B. (1985). "Health Case Study 35: The Effectiveness and Costs of Continuous Ambulatory Peritoneal Dialysis (CAPD)." Office of Technology Assessment, U.S. Congress. Washington, D.C.: U.S. Government Printing Office (September).

Steinberg, E. P., and Cohen, A. B. (1984). *Nuclear Magnetic Resonance Imaging Technology: A Clinical, Industrial, and Policy Analysis*. Health Technology Case Study #27. Prepared for the Office of Technology Assessment, U.S. Congress, OTA-HCS–27. Washington, D.C.: U.S. Government Printing Office (September).

Steinberg, E. P.; Sisk, J. E.; and Locke, K. E. (1985). "X-ray, CT, and Magnetic Resonance Imagers: Diffusion Patterns and Policy Issues." *New England Journal of Medicine* 313: 859–64.

Stern, R. S., and Epstein, A. M. (1985). "Institutional Responses to Prospective Payment Based on Diagnosis-Related Groups. Implications for Cost, Quality and Access." *New England Journal of Medicine* 312:621–27.

Teitelman, R. (1985). "Selective Surgery." *Forbes* 135, no. 8 (April): 75–76.

Thomas, L. (1971). "Notes of a Biology-watcher: The Technology of Medicine." *New England Journal of Medicine* 285:1366–68.

Thomas, L. (1974). "The Technology of Medicine." In *The Lives of a Cell*, L. Thomas, ed. New York: Viking Press.

Thompson, J. D. (1967). *Organizations in Action*. New York: McGraw-Hill, 11, 36.

Torrens, P. A. (1988). "Historical Evolution and Overview of Health Services in the United States." In *Introduction to Health Services*, S. J. Williams and P. R. Torrens, eds. 3d ed. New York: John Wiley & Sons, 3–31.

The 21st Congress of the European Dialysis and Transplant Association—European Renal Association. (1984). *Kidney International* 26:483–678.

Twiss, B. C. (1974). *Managing Technological Innovation*. London: Longman Group Ltd.

U.S. Congress. Senate. (1987). *The Health Care Innovation Act of 1987*. S–897.

U.S. Congress. Senate. Committee on Finance. (1972). Report to Accompany H.R. 1, The Social Security Amendments of 1972. Washington, D.C.: U.S. Government Printing Office. (September 26).

U.S. Congress. Senate. Committee on Finance. (1981). "End Stage Renal Disease Program Under Medicare." Washington, D.C.: U.S. Government Printing Office.

U.S. Congress. Senate. Committee on Finance. (1982a). "Proposed Prospective Reim-

bursement Rates for the End Stage Renal Disease Program under Medicare.''
Washington, D.C.: U.S. Government Printing Office (March).

U.S. Congress. Senate. Committee on Finance. (1982b). ''Proposed Prospective Payment
Rates for the End Stage Renal Disease Program.'' Hearings Before the Subcommittee on Health. Washington, D.C.: U.S. Government Printing Office (March
15).

U.S. General Accounting Office. (1982). Summary of GAO Testimony Before the Subcommittee on Health and the Environment (April).

Vallancien, G.; Aviles, J.; Munoz, A.; Charton, M.; and Brisset, J. M. (1988). ''Piezoelectric Extracorporeal Lithotripsy by Ultrashort Waves with the EDAPLTO1
Device.'' *Journal of Urology* 139, no. 4 (April): 689–94.

Vladeck, B. (1982). ''Controlling Costs by Changing Behavior: DRGs in New Jersey.''
Paper presented at the 100th annual meeting of the American Public Health Association, Montreal (November 17).

Vogel, E. (1979). *Japan as Number One: Lessons for America*. New York: Harper and
Row.

Volti, R. (1988). *Society and Technological Change*. New York: St. Martin's Press.

Wagner, J. L., and Krieger, M. (1980). ''The Price of Progress? Medical Technology
and Health Care Costs.'' *Journal of Contemporary Business* 9, no. 4 (Fall): 19–
33.

Weisbord, M. (1976). ''Why Organization Development Hasn't Worked (so far) In
Medical Centers.'' *Health Care Management Review* (Spring).

Whitcomb, M. E. (1988). ''Health Care Technology Acquisitions: Issues and Challenges.'' *Frontiers of Health Services Management* 4, no. 4 (Summer): 3–25.

Wild, R. (1987). ''Implications of Medicare Changes for Recovering Hospital Technology-Related Expenditures.'' Conference presentation. *Health Technology Adoption in a DRG Age*, Center for Technology and Policy, Boston University
(September).

Wilson, F. A., and Neuhauser, D. (1985). ''Ambulatory Care.'' *Health Services in the
United States*. Cambridge, Mass.: Ballinger, 43–60.

Index

About the Contributors

RONNA BORENSTEIN-LEVY, M.S., is Marketing Public Relations Manager, Medical Products Group, Hewlett-Packard Company. Her interests include medical technology, public health, and health care policy. She is the editor of Hewlett-Packard's quarterly magazine, *Advances for Medicine*.

HENRY P. BREHM, Ph.D., is Associate Professor of Sociology at the University of Maryland Baltimore County. In 1987, he directed the conference, "Health Technology Adoption in a DRG Age," at the Center for Technology and Policy, Boston University. His writings are in the areas of medical care organization and financing, aging, and disability, including coauthorship of a trilogy of books on social insurance policy issues subtitled: *From Social Problem to Federal Program*.

PAUL E. COAKLEY, JR., M.B.A., is Vice President, St. Agnes Hospital of the City of Baltimore, Inc. He is responsible for diagnostic and therapeutic services. His interests include health care administration, education, and medical technology.

JOHN L. FANTON, M.E.E., is Marketing Manager, Andover Division, Hewlett-Packard Company. He is interested in the area of instrumentation for the cardiovascular market. He is the author of several articles on instruments and marketing.

STAN N. FINKELSTEIN, M.D., is Director, Program of Health Policy and Management, Massachusetts Institute of Technology. He has written extensively in the area of medical technology decision-making and evaluation. He is the author of *Biomedical Innovation*.

DAVID T. GRIFFIN, Ph.D., is a principal with Hamilton/KSA, a health care consulting company that provides consulting services to medical products companies, hospitals, and physician groups. His expertise is in the clinical laboratory, diagnostic imaging, and cardiology products and services.

ALAN L. HILLMAN, M.D., M.B.A., is Assistant Professor of Health Care Systems and of Medicine, and Senior Fellow of the Leonard Davis Institute of Health Economics. His research focuses on how physicians make decisions to use health care technology and how those decisions can be influenced to create a safer and more equitable distribution of medical resources.

JOHN R. KIMBERLY, Ph.D., is Chairperson, Department of Management, and Professor of Management and Health Care Systems, the Wharton School of the University of Pennsylvania. He has written in the areas of organizational design and change and health policy management.

HENRY KRAKAUER, M.D., Ph.D., is Director, Office of Program Assessment and Information, Health Care Finance Administration. He is interested in and has written on the epidemiology of medical care in large populations, including the assessment of alternative technologies for the treatment of disease, the assessment of the quality of care, the use of quality measures in health care management, and evaluating and improving medical practice.

JAMES H. MAXWELL, Ph.D., is Visiting Scholar at the Massachusetts Institute of Technology and Research Assistant Professor at the State University of New York at Stony Brook. He has written on medical technology issues, examining the artificial heart, mechanical ventilation, renal dialysis, and biotechnology. He is completing a book on the evolution of Blue Cross and private health insurance.

SALLY BREWSTER MOULTON, M.A., is a doctoral student in sociology at Boston University. Her major interests and writings are in the areas of work and organizations, factors affecting scientific accomplishment, the impacts of technology on work and the labor force, and computer-based automation and labor relations in the construction equipment industry.

ROSS M. MULLNER, Ph.D., is Associate Professor and Director of the Center for Health Services Research, School of Public Health, University of Illinois at Chicago. He is the former Director, Hospital Research Center, Hospital Research and Educational Trust, American Hospital Association. His writings and interests include health care technology, hospital capital finance, hospital mergers, consolidations and closures, and the public policy implications of for-profit and not-for-profit hospitals.

SCOTT D. RAMSEY is a Ph.D. student in health care systems at the Wharton School of the University of Pennsylvania and a medical student at the University of Iowa. His research interests are alternative delivery systems, the evaluation and assessment of new medical technologies, and physician decision-making.

PAUL C. RETTIG, A.B., is Director of Government Relations, Mayo Clinic, Rochester, Minnesota. His interests include Medicare and health care finance issues. Formerly, he was Vice President for Health Care Policy of the Health Industry Manufacturers Association.

ROBERT F. RICH, Ph.D., is Director, Institute of Government and Public Affairs, University of Illinois. He is a professor of Political Science and acting head of Medical Humanities and Social Sciences in the College of Medicine on the Urbana-Champaign campus, and a professor of Health Resources Management at the School of Public Health on the Chicago campus.

JOYCE GRAHL RILEY, B.S.N., M.A., R.N., is Associate Director of the Health Science and Policy Program, University of Maryland Baltimore County. Her interests include education of health and social service providers and administrators concerning HIV/AIDS, and health care reimbursement as it affects hospital staffing patterns and introduction of technology.

LAURA E. ROPER, Ph.D., is a political science consultant. She has written on and is interested in primary health care service delivery, patient satisfaction, access and equity issues, and family planning issues.

VICTOR L. ROSENBERG, M.S.E. in Technology Policy, is a doctoral student in health care management at Boston University. He is the founder of Achiya Clinical Systems. He is interested in the health care organizational decision process.

STEPHEN R. ROSENTHAL, Ph.D., is Professor and Department Chairperson, Operations Management, School of Management, Boston University. His writings include works on the management of technological innovation and managing government operations.

HARVEY M. SAPOLSKY, Ph.D., is Professor of Public Policy and Organization at the Massachusetts Institute of Technology and has served as a consultant to several federal agencies and commissions. He has written in the health care field on the politics of product risks, decision-making in health planning and regulation, and federal health programs.

J. SANFORD SCHWARTZ, M.D., is Associate Professor of Medicine, Senior Fellow, Leonard Davis Institute of Health Economics, and Senior Scholar, Clinical Epidemiology Unit, University of Pennsylvania. His interests include evaluation of medical technology and adoption, diffusion and use practices, and medical decision-making. He has written on the diffusion and adoption of CT and MRI, and on human immunodeficiency virus test evaluation and strategy.

JAMES P. SHERBLOM, M.B.A., is Chairman and Chief Executive Officer, Transgenic Sciences, Inc., and President, Massachusetts Biotechnology Council.

NOREEN M. SUGRUE is a visiting lecturer at the Institute of Government and Public Affairs, University of Illinois. She is a Ph.D. student in Health Resources Management at the School of Public Health, University of Illinois.

MARY P. TAGGART, Ph.D., M.P.H., is Assistant Professor in the Graduate Program in Hospital and Health Administration at the University of Iowa. Her current interests include examining the post-PPS era in health care delivery with an emphasis on hospital closure.

PETER W. VAN ETTEN, M.B.A., is Executive Vice President and Chief Financial Officer, New England Medical Center.

DAVID G. WHITEIS, M.P.H., is currently completing his Ph.D. in the Health Planning and Policy Specialization of the Public Policy Analysis program at the University of Illinois at Chicago. His interests include hospital closure and its relationship to community economic development, and the public policy implications of the changing nature of U.S. health care delivery.